Did You Know ...

Clay (cosmetic) improves circulation, heals abrasions and removes toxins from the skin, replacing them with beneficial minerals . . .

Comfrey soothes sore throats, stops internal bleeding, heals stomach ulcers and normalizes excessive menstrual flow . . .

Goldenseal is one of nature's most versatile herbs, with powerful antiseptic, decongestant and anti-nausea applications. It is also used to treat skin irritations and sores, varicose veins, hemorrhoids and vaginal infections . . .

Olive oil heals and soothes skin irritations and injuries, lowers cholesterol, acts as a mild laxative, has antioxidant properties and is very effective in treating scalp disorders . . .

Rose, celebrated for its beauty and fragrance, is also an anti-inflammatory and antiseptic herb. . . .

—— ◂◦▸ ——

Discover the wonderful world of herbs in the must-have book chock full of easy, inexpensive recipes for everything from relief from common coughs to a safe, effective and absolutely wonderful herbal face-lift that takes years off your appearance without damaging your skin. It's all here and much more, in

—— ◂◦▸ ——

The Women's Home Remedy Kit

The Women's
Home Remedy Kit

Simple Recipes for Treating
Common Health Conditions

Maribeth Riggs

POCKET BOOKS

New York London Toronto Sydney Tokyo Singapore

An *Original* Publication of POCKET BOOKS

POCKET BOOKS, a division of Simon & Schuster Inc.
1230 Avenue of the Americas, New York, NY 10020

Copyright © 1995 by Maribeth Riggs

Library of Congress Cataloging-in-Publication Data

Riggs, Maribeth.
    The women's home remedy kit : simple recipes for treating common health conditions / Maribeth Riggs.
        p.   cm.
    ISBN: 0-671-89806-X
    1. Herbs—Therapeutic use.   2. Women—Health and hygiene.
I. Title.
RM666.H33R54   1995
615'.321—dc20   95-14004
                                                                        CIP

First Pocket Books trade paperback printing October 1995

10 9 8 7 6 5 4 3 2 1

POCKET and colophon are registered trademarks of
Simon & Schuster Inc.

Cover design by

Interior illustrations by Elizabeth Garsonnin

Printed in the U.S.A.

Dedication

——— ◄◦► ———

This book is dedicated to my family—past, present, and future—and to my parents, Guy Wadsworth Quire Riggs and Selma Helene Hubka Riggs.

Acknowledgments

——— ◄◦► ———

I would like to express my sincere thanks and appreciation to Rita Aero, Candace Fuhrman, Elizabeth Garsonnin, and Claire Zion for their help and guidance throughout the preparation of this book.

Contents

—◇—

Introduction   xi

Part 1
Key Herbs and Ingredients

Almond   3
Aloe Vera   5
Barley   7
Beeswax   9
Black Cherry Extract   10
Clay (Cosmetic)   12
Comfrey   14
Dong Quai   16
Echinacea   18
Ginger   20
Goldenseal   22
Lavender   24

Contents

Lemon   26
Oats   28
Olive   30
Peppermint   32
Pennyroyal   34
Plantain   36
Rose   38
Rosemary   40
Slippery Elm   41
Valerian Root   43
Witch Hazel   45

Part 2

Symptoms and Recipes

Acne   51
Anemia   53
Arthritis   55
Backaches   57
Bladder Infections   59
Breast Tenderness   61
Burns (minor)   63
Cold Sores   65
Constipation   67
Coughs   69
Cuts (minor)   71
Dandruff   73
Diarrhea   75

Contents

Dry or Damaged Hair 77

Dry Skin 79

Eye Strain 81

Foot Problems 83

Hair Loss 85

Hangover 87

Head Congestion 89

Headaches 91

Hemorrhoids 93

Hot Flashes 95

Insomnia 97

Liver Spots 99

Menstrual Cramping 101

Morning Sickness 103

Muscle Tension 105

Nausea 107

Nervous Tension 109

Oily Hair 111

Oily Skin 113

Sinusitis 115

Skin Rashes 117

Sore Throats 119

Stomachaches 121

Stretch Marks 123

Swollen Glands 125

Vaginal Infections 127

Varicose Veins 129

Water Retention 131

Wrinkles 133

Contents

Part 3
Source Guide

Some Recommendations 139
Wholesale and Retail Mail-Order Outlets 141
Herbal Publications and Newsletters 144

Introduction

————— ◀◇▶ —————

Like many women, I fit physical checkups in between child care, jobs, relationships, dinners, and the laundry. When I find myself sick, sore, achy, or injured in some way, I want relief and I want it fast. Western allopathic medicine often has the answer, and that is why I consider myself lucky to have great health insurance and a very nice family-practice doctor.

But just as often, for many of my minor aches and pains, I turn to inexpensive and effective herbal remedies. Herbs are a natural complement to modern medicine as they strengthen the immune system and provide underlying nourishment and support for the healing process. They give you the opportunity to decide why, when, and how to develop your own personal health-care products. You can indulge yourself and try hundreds of herbs and recipe combinations, or you can enjoy a few tried-and-true favorites year after year. If you wish to combine the use of herbs with medical treatment, consult with your physician beforehand.

Introduction

When I first started choosing herbs and recipes as part of my own and my children's health care, I found myself overwhelmed by the amount of information available. There were so many choices to make, not only regarding what herbs to use, but their combinations as well. I started learning all I could about herbs, through independent study and by obtaining a Certificate of Herbalism from the California School of Herbal Studies, which was, at that time, directed by the inspirational Rosemary Gladstar. Over the years, my initial trial-and error approach became an organized system, linking symptoms to their appropriate herbal cures and diet/lifestyle changes. The recipes in this book reflect this system, which is based in large part on economy, simplicity, practicality, safety, and need.

In planning *The Women's Home Remedy Kit,* I thought of forty over-drugged or under-cured symptoms that women and their doctors must deal with. Many of these common, chronic symptoms leave doctors—and consequently their patients—at a loss, either because the drugs prescribed don't work or because the side effects produced when they are used are undesirable. For these conditions, including recurring vaginal infections, skin rashes, cramps, insomnia, and morning sickness, to name just a few, beneficial herbs (and the information contained in this book) can make the healing difference.

For all the recipes in this book I have compiled a list of just twenty-three herbs to choose from, most of which are probably already in your kitchen. These are herbs I've kept on hand for every household emergency, as well nonemergency and beauty treatments, for the past twenty years. They are completely safe to use when prepared and taken according to the recipe instructions. Many can be used singly or in combination with only one or two other herbs with excellent results. All may be found in health-food stores, and many are found in any supermarket. My final selection criterion is expense. All of the listed ingredients, even the exotic dong quai, are inexpensive. When you find yourself selecting from nature's limitless array of healing herbs, remember that safety, effectiveness, and affordability are always the qualities to rely on.

Part 1

———◦◊◦———

Key Herbs and Ingredients

Almond

Prunus amygdalus

Hulled almonds are approximately 1 inch long and oval shaped, with a rough, brown surface. Almond oil is light yellow and has little or no smell. Hardy, drought-resistant almond trees can grow up to 20 feet high, producing lovely, fragrant pink blossoms seasonally. Almonds are cultivated as a food crop in California, Israel, southern Europe, and all around the Mediterranean. They grow wild in the Jamaican islands, where the blooming flowers produce an intoxicating perfume.

Almond oil is high in vitamin E and is an herbal emollient, which means that it nourishes and soothes dry or rashy skin. A paste made of ground almonds has a cleansing, softening, and mild bleaching action

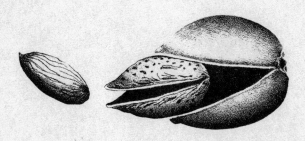

on the skin, making it an extremely popular ingredient in many cosmetic preparations.

Recent research has revealed almond oil's value as a cholesterol-lowering agent when used in the diet in place of saturated fats. Additionally, a tablespoon of almond oil can soothe the digestive tract and relieve the symptoms of gastritis, nausea, and cramps. Almond butter makes a delicious low-fat alternative to peanut butter.

Almonds are available fresh or as an oil extract. Fresh hulled almonds are available in health-food and grocery stores. Do not buy skinless, slivered, or blanched almonds for the purposes of this book. Almond oil is available in pharmacies but this product is highly refined and is not recommended. Purchase almond oil in bath and cosmetic shops or in health-food stores.

Store almond oil in a dark, airtight jar and discard it after six months. Fresh almonds keep well for approximately one month in an airtight plastic bag or jar in a pantry or cupboard.

Aloe Vera

——— ‹o› ———

Aloe vera

The aloe is a succulent cactus with long, fleshy, spine-edged leaves. The plant produces a 5-foot flower stalk, with droopy orange flowers growing from the top. There are almost two hundred varieties of this plant growing throughout the world, but the aloe vera (meaning "true aloe") is the one most widely used for healing and cosmetics. The broad leaves contain a greenish, translucent, salve-like juice that is emollient, or nourishing and soothing, to the skin. This juice is used in skin creams, lip balms, hair dressings, and as a natural burn remedy.

In many tropical countries, aloe vera juice is used externally for ringworm infestation and internally to expel intestinal parasites. In both Europe and America, the juice of the aloe vera plant is sold as a tonic and laxative. The commercial gel can be applied to minor cuts and burns or insect bites and, in diluted form, used as a wash for tired or infected eyes.

Many people prefer using raw aloe vera juice from a plant growing at home. However, the raw juice can cause allergic reactions and mild burns, especially if used on tender or irritated skin. Commercial aloe vera gel is dehydrated aloe juice reconstituted with water and a preservative for freshness. I recommend using the bottled gel, which is mild, yet effective.

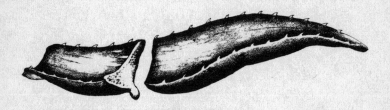

Aloe is a perennial plant found wild in East and South Africa and in the southwestern United States. It is cultivated in the West Indies and other tropical areas.

Aloe vera gel is available in health-food stores, bath shops, and pharmacies. Keep the gel refrigerated after opening and discard any leftover gel after six months.

Barley

—◄○►—

Hordeum vulgare

Barley is an annual grass that is widely cultivated as a food grain. The barley plant grows up to 3 feet high, the bristly barley grains sprouting at the top of the stalk. Removing the outer hull of the barley grain exposes the white, oval-shaped kern, which is approximately ¼ inch long. Because of its shiny-white color and shape, this product is called "pearled barley."

Barley was once consumed by the ancient Romans to promote potency and vigor and is still consumed today as a healthful breakfast food. Vast quantities of roasted barley grains are used in the United States to flavor beer, and the spent barley grains are then used as animal fodder.

When pearled barley is cooked, it becomes mucilaginous, which means that it releases a gel-like substance. This substance is a well-known and nutritious thickener for soups and stews, and its easy digestibility makes it a good remedy for gastrointestinal problems. The chemical constituents of barley, when taken as a tea, in muffins, or as an oil in capsules, block the liver's manufacture of cholesterol, thus helping to ward off heart disease and terol, thus helping to ward off heart disease and possibly cancer. Barley water taken internally acts as a mild diuretic. Used externally, barley water is an excellent wash for skin irritations.

Barley can be found chopped, rolled, unhulled, or pearled in grocery and health-food stores. Barley grits, flakes, cracked barley, and barley flour are also available in health-food stores. For the purposes of this book, organic pearled barley is preferred, though commercial pearled barley is effective and more easily found.

Store pearled barley in an airtight jar or plastic bag in a cupboard, away from heat and light. Discard the barley after one month.

Beeswax

——— ◄◦► ———

Beeswax is produced by honeybees, for the purpose of storing honey and larvae, and also to serve as a structural support for the hive. This propolis-rich substance is fashioned into a sturdy, ladder-like system of containers known as the honeycomb. Fresh honeycomb is a delicious treat, as raw beeswax is edible and contains the delectable honey.

Beeswax is used as a medium for ointments and salves, and in home canning and candlemaking. Beeswax candles burn long and bright and fill the room with a honey-like fragrance. Scented beeswax candles and pomanders were considered a rare and expensive luxury in Colonial times.

Processed beeswax is usually a deep golden brown in color. If the beeswax has not been processed and is part of a honeycomb, it will be made up of many regularly spaced hexagonal chambers.

Beeswax can be found in the form of raw honeycomb or it can be found in jars or formed into blocks for use in candlemaking and home canning. If you do not live near an apiary (a bee farm, where honey is produced) go to the nearest health-food store or craft shop. If you buy the beeswax in candle

form, be sure it is composed of pure beeswax, with
no scented oils added. Be careful to avoid the wick
when grating the beeswax candle for adding to ointments and salves. An unscented, highly processed
beeswax is available in pharmacies, but it resembles
paraffin and is not as aesthetically pleasing as the
unprocessed product.

Black Cherry Extract

Cerasus vulgaris

Black cherries grow abundantly throughout Europe
and the eastern United States. The trees grow to 30
feet or more in height, producing seasonal fragrant
white flowers. The purplish-black fruit, approximately 1 inch in diameter, hangs in clusters and
has a sweet, slightly pungent taste when fully ripe.
Black cherries are a popular ingredient in jams, jel-
lies, juices, and syrups.

Besides providing delicious fruit, cherry trees
have other medicinal uses. Wild cherry bark (*Prunus serotina*) is used as an ingredient in cough
syrup and stomach bitters, while the bark of the
Virginia cherry tree (*Prunus virginiana*) provides a
gel-like substance useful in herbal hair conditioners
and other cosmetic preparations.

Black cherries have been used for centuries in the

Western world to treat gout, iron deficiency, rheumatism, constipation, and, because of their tonic effect on the nervous system, stress and anxiety. They are specific for symptoms indicating lowered immune resistance and vitamin deficiency, such as anemia, bleeding gums, or fatigue. Cherries were once believed to possess magical rejuvenating powers, probably because of the high amounts of iron, vitamin C, vitamin B, and raw fructose they contain.

Black cherries are available fresh, in juice form, or dried in bulk. Organic black cherry extract is available in health-food stores and some grocery stores. Select a brand that has no added preservatives or sweeteners. Refrigerate the extract after opening and discard any leftovers after six months.

Clay (Cosmetic)

Since prehistoric times, clay has been known to humans and animals as a universal healing agent. Many mammal species cover themselves in mud to protect their skin and to relieve pain and irritation. Humankind flatters itself to think that a mud bath at a luxurious spa is far removed from an African elephant's favorite riverbottom wallow, but both species seek the healing power of clay, and for the same reasons. Clay or mud packs improve circulation, heal abrasions, and remove toxins from the skin, replacing them with beneficial minerals. The drying power of clay also tightens and tones the skin, increasing sex appeal by making it firmer and younger-looking.

Because of its high concentration of minerals and its ability to draw flesh together as it dries, clay is applied topically to burned or scarred tissue, and in the case of sprains and broken bones. Today's calcium-rich plaster cast evolved from the old-fashioned use of wet clay and splints for setting fractures and sprains. Clay packs have also been used to draw venom from snake and insect bites and to dissolve tumors, calcium deposits, and cysts.

A paste of cosmetic clay applied to your face absorbs excess oil from the top layer of skin while removing dead, dry cells. As the mask dries, the tightening action stimulates circulation and makes your skin glow. I recommend the use of French green clay, which is highly refined and rich in mineral and vegetable nutrients, yet balanced for all skin types and conditions. Kaolin, bentonite, fuller's earth, and zinc oxide are the most common ingredients found in commercial clay mask formulas. Though useful in cases of oily or acned skin, these commercial ingredients can be too dehydrating for dry or mature complexions.

Dry French green clay is available in bath shops, department stores, health-food stores, and through wholesale and retail herb outlets. Store the dry clay in a dark, air- and watertight jar, away from heat and light, for up to a year.

Comfrey

Symphytum officinale

Fresh comfrey leaves are dark green, thick, fleshy, and fuzzy-feeling to the touch. Dried comfrey leaves are a darker green color, with a mellow, musty smell. The fresh root is dark brown on the outside and stark white on the inside, with a sharp, earthy odor.

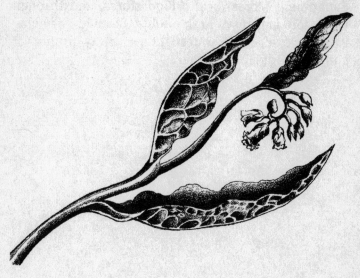

Comfrey

Comfrey grows wild in the United States and Europe. The whole plant can be used—the root for medicine and the leaves for tea or as a fresh salad green.

Comfrey is widely used as a healing herb. Its versatility makes it useful for healing burns, severe rashes, skin eruptions, cuts, and scrapes, and a plaster made from comfrey can be applied to the breasts and other areas of the body to provide relief from tenderness and soreness. Comfrey contains large amounts of calcium and allantoin, making it an excellent remedy for muscle, skin, and bone disorders. A decoction of comfrey root is used to soothe sore throats, stop internal bleeding, heal stomach ulcers, and normalize excessive menstrual flow.

Dried comfrey root is available chopped into small pieces or ground into a powder. It can also be found in tablet form or in capsules. Dried leaves, root pieces, tablets, and capsules are available in health-food stores and through wholesale and retail herb outlets. Comfrey can be grown easily in a pot or garden.

Dried comfrey leaf stores well in a dark, airtight jar for one month. Comfrey root pieces are hardier and may be kept in an airtight plastic bag or clear glass jar for up to six months.

Dong Quai

—◄◊►—

Angelica sinensis

A close cousin to American and European angelica, dong quai enjoys a reputation as the "female ginseng." The dong quai plant grows to 3 feet in height and has graceful, spreading leaves. The medicinal part is the thick, ivory-colored root, which takes many interesting shapes and forms.

Dong quai grows well at high altitudes and loves cool, damp places. It is native to western and northern China, and is cultivated there as well as in the United States and Europe.

Dong quai is used for a wide variety of female disorders, including irregular menstruation, painful menstrual cramps, and discomfort due to premenstrual syndrome. The herb restores normal periodic flow after the discontinuation of birth-control pills and relieves hot flashes and other symptoms associated with menopause. Dong quai is high in vitamins and minerals, including vitamins A, B_{12}, and E, and is used to treat insomnia, high blood pressure, and anemia in both sexes. Though it contains no plant estrogens, it nourishes the blood and has a mild stimulating and cleansing effect upon the liver, the organ responsible for regulating much of the body's hormone production.

Dong quai is available in whole root form, dried and chopped into pieces, sliced and cured, and as a powder, tincture, syrup, or extract. It is available in health-food stores and through wholesale and retail herb outlets. The highest-quality dong quai root is found in Chinese pharmacies and herb shops.

Dried dong quai root pieces and powder are best stored in a dark, airtight jar for up to six months. Tinctures, syrups, and extracts should be kept in a dark closet, away from heat and light. Refrigerate syrups or extracts after opening for up to two months. Because of its ability to relax uterine tissue, this herb is not recommended for pregnant women.

Echinacea

Echinacea augustifolia or *E. purpurea*

Echinacea enjoys a variety of folk names, including Sampson root and purple coneflower. The American settlers were introduced to this native American herb by the Sioux and other Great Plains tribes, who used it to draw venom from snake bites.

Echinacea is a perennial plant growing from the prairie states northward to Pennsylvania. The bristly stem has hairy leaves and startling purple flowers, which bloom from June through October. The medicinal part is the root stock, which dries to a dull grayish-brown color.

This popular herb has been thoroughly researched in the Western scientific community and is considered an herbal antibiotic among herbalists in America and Europe. When taken internally, echinacea helps the body to fight invading organisms on a cellular level, and the same bacteria-fighting properties prevent infection when applied externally to wounds, which explains its well-deserved reputation as an immune-system support. The root is also a blood-purifyer, useful for acne, boils, rashes, and other symptoms indicating contaminants in the blood. Powdered echinacea root can be applied directly to abscessed teeth, bedsores, or slow-healing wounds for quick relief. In tincture form, it brings down fevers, stops colds and flus from advancing, and helps settle digestive disorders.

The dried, powdered root has a powerful pungent smell, which indicates its strength and freshness. Echinacea root is available chopped into pieces or ground into a powder. It can also be found in tablet form, as a tincture, or in capsules in health-food stores and through retail and wholesale herb outlets.

Dried echinacea root pieces, capsules, tablets, and powder store well for up to four months in a dark, airtight jar. Tinctures last for years, but should be stored in a closet or cupboard, away from heat and light.

Ginger

Zingiber officinale

The ginger plant grows to a height of 4 feet and produces a simple, leafy stem and spike-shaped white flowers with purple and yellow spots. The tan-colored knobby root has a strong aroma and is popular as a medicine and culinary spice and flavoring agent.

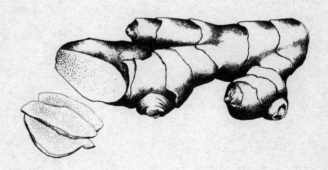

Ginger is native to China and India, and it is extensively cultivated in the West Indies, India, and Africa. The first bulk imports of ginger were brought to the western hemisphere centuries ago by the Dutch East India Company and were quickly snapped up to flavor rum, brandy, syrups, and cordials.

Ginger

Hot ginger tea brings on a profuse sweat and has a warming effect upon the lungs and gastrointestinal tract, making it a good cold and flu remedy. It is also an antinauseant that can be safely used for morning sickness, upset stomach, infant colic, and intestinal gas. Applied locally as a compress or liniment, ginger root brings blood to a congested joint or muscle, relieving the pain of arthritis, backaches, muscle tension, and swelling. Because of its ability to stimulate circulation throughout the entire body, it is an excellent remedy for headaches, hangovers, and water retention. Ginger root clears the sinuses and lungs when used in facials and baths.

Fresh, whole, and powdered ginger root are popular culinary ingredients and can be found in supermarkets. Dried, bulk powder, and essential oil of ginger can be found in health-food stores, through wholesale and retail herb outlets, and in Chinese pharmacies and herb shops.

Fresh ginger keeps well in the refrigerator but should be discarded when it starts to shrivel, usually after two weeks. Ginger powder and dried ginger pieces should be kept in dark, airtight jars, for no longer than four months.

Goldenseal

——— ◆◇◆ ———

Hydrastis canadensis

Goldenseal root is bright yellow when fresh, and a deep, dark golden color when powdered and dried. Growing up to 9 inches high, it produces a solitary white- or rose-colored flower and seasonal red fruits that resemble raspberries, which explains its folk name, "ground raspberry."

Goldenseal is native to North America and grows as a creeping perennial in cool, shaded areas throughout the Northeast and as far west as Ohio. The Native Americans of the northeastern United States gave goldenseal root, along with corn and tobacco, as gifts to the Pilgrims and taught them to use it as medicine and as a dye for cloth and leather.

Goldenseal is one of nature's most versatile herbs. It is a powerful antiseptic, and is used internally to cleanse and disinfect the liver, lymph, and bloodstream, to decongest the lungs and sinuses, and to relieve nausea. Used externally as a wash, douche, or liniment, goldenseal is specific for skin irritations and sores, varicose veins, hemorrhoids, and vaginal infections. Goldenseal stimulates the liver and, in tea or tincture form, is excellent for restoration of the period after the discontinuation of birth-control pills or for regulation of hormones during menopause. This herb has a stimulating effect on the lymphatic and circulatory systems and must be taken in carefully measured doses. Do not use this herb if you have high blood pressure or if you are pregnant.

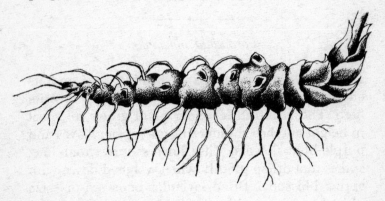

Goldenseal is available as a fresh or dried root, chopped into pieces, and powdered in bulk. It is also found in tablet form, as a tincture, and in capsules. Goldenseal products are available in health-food stores and through wholesale and retail herb outlets.

Powdered goldenseal root and dried root pieces store well in a dark, airtight jar for up to four months. Tinctures last for years and should be kept in a cupboard, away from heat and light.

Lavender

━◄◊►━

Lavandula officinalis

Lavender, with its multiple healing uses and its eternally soothing fragrance is, by far, my favorite herb. The beautiful lavender plant grows to 2 feet in height and has shimmering gray-green leaves and purple-blue flowers. The flowers grow from long spikes that droop prettily when weighed down with spring blossoms. Dried lavender buds are the size of barley grains, with a dark purple color.

The familiar, pungent smell of lavender graces any herb garden, from the formal châteaus and estates of Europe to simple cottage hedges and paths. Lavender is native to southern Europe, and it grows wild around the Mediterranean, in southern England, and along the western coast of the United States. It came to America with the Pilgrim women and was planted in kitchen gardens as an ornamental and medicinal herb.

When used as an inhalant, lavender oil relieves depression and insomnia. Lavender oil mixed with water or alcohol makes an antiseptic wash for skin rashes and irritations. When added to a hot bath, lavender oil or buds relieve sore feet, tense muscles, and frayed nerves. Diarrhea, nausea, and headaches respond well to a few drops of lavender oil added to hot water and taken as tea. Diluted with olive or almond oil, essential oil of lavender can be massaged into the skin to fade stretch marks, speed the closing of wounds and scar tissue, and relieve varicose veins. Lavender oil is a popular commercial ingredient in perfumes, cosmetics, and hair preparations.

Dried lavender buds and essential oil of lavender can be found in health-food stores and through wholesale and retail herb outlets. Lavender is easily grown in a garden.

Dried lavender buds can be kept in airtight jars or plastic bags for up to four months. Essential oil of lavender should be kept in dark, airtight jars at room temperature, away from heat and light, for no more than six months.

Lemon

Citrus limon

Lemon is a popular fruit tree, grown in warm climates throughout the United States, particularly in California and Florida. The familiar lemon is oval-shaped, approximately 4 inches in length, and distinctively yellow in color. The juice and rind of the fruit produce a sharp citrus aroma.

The juice of the lemon fruit and the oil produced in its rind are used medicinally and cosmetically. Lemon juice is the chief ingredient in lemonade, a cooling and liver-cleansing hot-weather beverage.

Lemon juice is antiseptic and refrigerant, meaning it cools and disinfects inflammations and wounds. Powdered lemon peel was carried by World War I medics, who packed it into wounds to stop bleeding and reduce the risk of infection. This "field antibiotic" is still useful today to reduce the risk of food poisoning. When lemon juice is sprinkled onto shellfish, 95 percent of all the bacteria contained therein disappear within fifteen minutes, which explains the ubiquitous wedge of lemon when seafood is served. Lemon juice is highly acidic and has a mild bleaching action on liver spots, freckles, and scars. The juice taken internally reinforces the immune system by detoxifying the liver, gastrointestinal tract, and urinary tract, making it a good remedy for colds and flu, water retention, and bladder infections. Lemon juice tightens and disinfects the soft tissues of the mouth and throat, relieving bleeding gums, sore throats, and canker sores. Diluted lemon juice makes an excellent final rinse for skin and scalp.

Juice your own lemons for the purposes of this book. Buy organic or unwaxed lemons, available in grocery stores, health-food stores, or at organic farm stands. Scrub them well if you wish to use the peels. Lemons store well in the refrigerator but should be discarded after two weeks.

Oats

--- ◀◦▶ ---

Avena sativa

The oat plant is a grass that grows from 2 to 4 feet high. The stalks, leaves, and berries are used for medicine, food, and animal fodder. Oat berries, slightly larger than rice grains, are a rich, dark brown color. Oat straw, the dried green stalk and leaves of the oat plant, is pale yellow in color.

Oats have been cultivated as a food crop in Europe and America for centuries and are used primarily as a breakfast food. Because of its digestibility, it is also used as a nourishing food for convalescents.

Oats are specific for repairing frazzled nerve endings, as they contain B vitamins and a rich supply of minerals, including calcium, iron, phosphorous, and silica. Oats in tincture or tea form are recommended for insomnia, anxiety, or nervous exhaustion due to hormonal imbalances or prolonged stress, and for treating external stress-related symptoms, including herpes outbreaks, shingles, and hives. Organic oatmeal and oat bran, when eaten on a daily basis, significantly lower serum cholesterol levels in the body, reducing the risk of heart attack and high blood pressure. Because of its digestibility and high fiber content, cereals and teas containing oats are indicated for morning sickness, gastroenteritis, and constipation. Scars, acne, and skin irritations respond well to baths, soaps, facials, and compresses containing whole or ground oats.

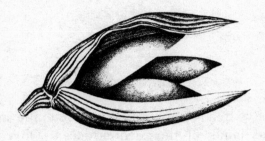

Dried oat berries are available rolled, chopped into small pieces, or ground to a meal. Because many nutrients are lost in commercial processing, I recommend purchasing organic, rolled oat berries from health-food stores and through wholesale and retail herb outlets for medicinal, dietary, and cosmetic use.

Dried, rolled oat berries can be stored in a dark, airtight jar or in an airtight plastic bag for up to a month. Oat tinctures may be kept in a cupboard, away from heat and light, for years.

Olive

———— ◄◦► ————

Olea europaea

The olive tree is an evergreen, native to the ancient biblical lands of the Mediterranean. Olive trees grow to 25 feet in height, producing a hard yellow wood covered with gray-green bark. Olive trees produce seasonal fragrant white flowers and the familiar olive fruit, which is eaten as a food and processed for its oil.

Olive trees are cultivated in tropical and warm climates. Beside the fruit and its oil, the leaves and inner bark of olive trees are used in teas to reduce fever and calm the nerves.

Olive oil is demulcent and emollient, which means that it heals and soothes skin irritations and injuries. Pure olive oil can be applied externally to burns, bruises, insect bites, sprains, and itchy rashes to relieve pain and discomfort. Its most common use is as a base for ointments, massage oils, and liniments. When taken internally, olive oil dramatically lowers cholesterol levels, soothes the gastrointestinal tract, and acts as a mild laxative. Recent research has revealed olive oil's antioxidant qualities, and it has been used to treat abnormal cell growth in cancer patients and to retard the aging process. A hair oil made of olive oil and essential oil of rosemary is good for scalp disorders and hair loss.

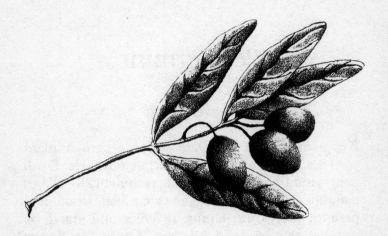

Olive oil is available in any grocery store, but I recommend using only fresh, dark green, extra-virgin olive oil for medicinal purposes. This type of olive oil is available in Mediterranean-style delicatessens, health-food stores, and gourmet food stores. Highly processed, odorless olive oil is sold in pharmacies, but I do not recommend its use.

Olive oil should be stored in an airtight jar in a cupboard, away from heat and light. Discard leftover olive oil after six months.

Peppermint

◄◉►

Mentha piperita

Peppermint is a familiar, creeping garden plant with dark green, pointed, serrated leaves. Fresh peppermint leaves exude a characteristically sharp, menthol aroma when broken or mashed. Dried peppermint leaves are fainter in color and smell, as most of the essential oils are lost in the drying process.

Peppermint is native to Europe and the United States and is cultivated and found wild in both countries. It is used as a flavoring agent in chewing gum, toothpaste, and cordials. Its old-fashioned popularity in alcoholic beverages gave it the folk name "brandymint."

Versatile peppermint is a carminative, which means that it aids digestion, and an expectorant, or an herb that promotes the discharge of mucous from the respiratory passages. Peppermint in the form of a tea, tincture, or cordial helps control nausea, morning sickness, headache, and hangovers. As an inhalant, peppermint oil can be used to relieve head and lung congestion, insomnia, and nervous tension. Because of its unique ability to dilate and then constrict blood vessels when applied to the skin, it is a popular ingredient in facials, liniments, baths, and massage oils. Peppermint is an excellent coolant and can be used internally as a tea or tincture and externally as a spray to relieve hot flashes and fevers.

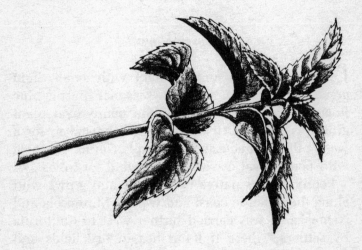

Dried peppermint is a popular culinary ingredient and can be found fresh in supermarkets. Essential oil of peppermint can be found in health-food stores and through wholesale and retail herb outlets. Peppermint is easily grown in a garden.

Fresh peppermint leaves can be stored in the refrigerator for up to a week. Dried leaves store well in dark, airtight jars for up to four months. Essential oil of peppermint should be kept at room temperature, away from heat and light.

Pennyroyal

—◄○►—

Hedeoma pulegioides

Pennyroyal is an annual plant with small, light green, serrated leaves and seasonal purple-blue flowers. The single stalk of the pennyroyal plant grows as high as 18 inches. Easily mistaken for a weed, the characteristic champhor-mint scent of wild pennyroyal carries on the wind for miles.

Pennyroyal is native to America and grows wild along the Atlantic coast and west to Minnesota and Nebraska. It was carried further west to California by settlers, where it flourishes in dry fields and open woods.

Hot pennyroyal tea promotes a sweat when taken internally, and should be taken at the onset of a cold or flu. Applied externally, pennyroyal massage oil relieves the pain and discomfort of menstrual cramps by bringing circulation to the pelvic area and stimulating uterine contractions. When added to a bath or facial steam, pennyroyal's strong aroma decongests the sinuses and lungs, relieving coughs and head congestion. Because of its ability to stimulate circulation and relieve congestion, it is an excellent external remedy for swollen glands. Pennyroyal tea can be used as a wash to relieve insect bites and other skin irritations. The essential oil of pennyroyal is used commercially in insecticides and flea repellents.

Pennyroyal is available chopped and dried or as an oil extract. The distilled oil is far more concentrated than the leaves and is poisonous if taken internally. Use it externally only and under the supervision of a medical herbalist or holistic physician. The dried, chopped leaves are available in health-food stores and through wholesale and retail herb outlets. Pennyroyal can be easily grown in a garden. This herb is not recommended for use by pregnant women.

Dried pennyroyal leaf stores well in a dark, airtight jar for up to four months.

Plantain

Plantago lanceolata and P. major

Plantain leaves have two general shapes, spear- or lance-shaped (*lanceolata*) and broad-leafed (*major*). Both varieties grow up to 18 inches high and produce a spiky blossom stalk with greenish-white flowers at the tip. Dried plantain is dark green, with a mild musty smell.

Plantain is a humble herb, growing in abandoned lots, yards, and roadsides wherever the climate is temperate. In early times, plantain was the only edible herb certain to be found by travelers walking the roads, earning it the folk names "soldier's herb" and "way bread." Unfortunately, plantain is now regarded as an unattractive weed and is often sprayed or dug up on public and private lands.

Plantain is demulcent and astringent: that is, it heals and disinfects skin injuries and irritations. It is specific for healing and regenerating burned skin. When used as an ingredient in massage oils or ointments, plantain reduces swelling and congestion, and is indicated for tender, aching breasts, hemorrhoids, and sprains. Plantain, soothing to mucous-lined surfaces, is a good ingredient in douche formulas. Tea made from dried leaves relieves gastrointestinal problems, and the extracted juice of fresh leaves can be used to rid the body of intestinal parasites. Plantain tea is a mild diuretic and can be taken to relieve water retention.

Plantain grows wild in waste places all over the world, but you should harvest it only where you are certain it has not been sprayed. Dried plantain is available chopped and in tablet form in health-food stores and through wholesale and retail herb outlets. It is probably growing in your yard or garden right now.

Fresh plantain can be stored in the refrigerator for up to a week. Dried leaves store well in dark, airtight jars for up to four months.

Rose

◄◦►

Rosa spp.

The lovely rose has inspired romantic verses, songs, and works of art through the ages. Roses have numerous delicate, velvet-soft petals that surround yellow anthers in the center of the flower. Wild roses are smaller and thornier than garden varieties, but have a stronger fragrance. Dried rosebuds and petals are dull red or pink and withered-looking.

Roses are native to the Middle East and temperate zones in China. Their beauty, fragrance, and medicinal qualities captivated early explorers, who brought back seedlings and grafts for planting in western gardens. There are now more than one hundred varieties of rose throughout the northern hemisphere. Damask rose (*Rosa damascena*) and Provence rose (*Rosa gallica*) are the original roses of pharmacy.

Roses exude a powerful fragrance, which is useful as a restorative and for relieving depression and insomnia. Rose is an anti-inflammatory and antiseptic herb and is taken internally to relieve gastrointestinal problems, liver congestion, and inflammations of the bladder. The ancient Romans prevented drunkenness by inhaling rose essence from garlands worn around their necks, and a dose of rose water or rose tea is specific for relieving the nausea and tiredness of hangovers. Rose oil and distilled rose water are used externally as an astringent ingredient in washes, oils, and ointments formulated for dry hair and skin.

Roses are cultivated and grow wild in temperate zones throughout the United States. Red and pink rose petals may be harvested for rose water, but be sure they have not been sprayed. I recommend purchasing culinary-grade rose water, which is available through Middle Eastern delicatessens and health-food stores, for the recipes in this book. Keep the rose water at room temperature, away from heat and light.

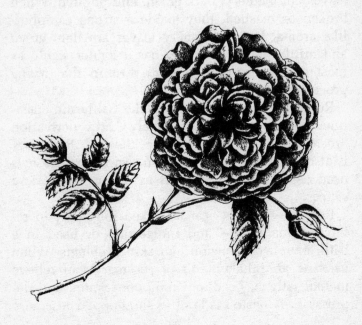

Rosemary

Rosmarinus officinalis

Rosemary is a woody, evergreen shrub with seasonal, delicate blue flowers. It grows prolifically, often crowding out nearby plants. Fresh rosemary leaves are leathery, dark green, and pointed. When broken or mashed, they exude a strong camphorlike aroma. Dried rosemary leaves are light green and brittle. Dried rosemary has a lighter smell, as most of the essential oils are lost in the drying process.

Rosemary grows wild along the California coastline, which explains its lovely Latin derivation "rosmarinus," meaning "dew of the sea." Rosemary is also native to Mediterranean regions, where it is used as a popular addition in soups, stews, and sauces.

Rosemary leaf tea can be taken internally to relieve stomachaches and indigestion or used in a bath for muscle tension and skin problems. When used as an inhalant, oil of rosemary can relieve mental fatigue, head and lung congestion, and depression. A paste made of fresh chopped rosemary leaves is excellent as an herbal skin and foot rub. The volatile oils contained in the rosemary plant are also used pharmaceutically and commercially in medicines, room fresheners, and insect repellents.

Dried rosemary is a popular culinary ingredient and can be found in supermarkets. Essential oil of rosemary can be found in health-food stores and through wholesale and retail herb outlets. Rosemary can be grown easily in a garden.

Fresh rosemary leaves may be stored in the refrigerator for up to a week. Dried leaves store well in dark, airtight jars for up to four months.

Slippery Elm

——— ◄◦► ———

Ulmus fulva

The noble elm is planted as an ornamental tree throughout the eastern United States, especially in urban areas, where it beautifies and shades city sidewalks and streets. American elm trees grow to 50 feet in height, exhibiting a rough-textured outer bark and downy leaves. The part used medicinally is the inner bark, which is shaved, dried, and ground to a powder. This powder is soft and beige-pink in color and has a sweet, aromatic fragrance.

The high level of mucilage contained in powdered elm bark is what gives the herb its folk name, slippery elm. The mucilage is released when the powder is boiled, creating a gel-like pabulum. This pabulum is easily digested and was once prescribed as a nutritious food for invalids and as a remedy for constipation. Slippery elm tea coats and soothes the gastrointestinal tract, relieving diarrhea, morning sickness, heartburn, and acid indigestion. The pabulum can also be used to lessen the discomfort of ulcers and colitis. The powder or paste can be applied to blemished skin, minor wounds, or rashes to soothe irritation and promote healing, and for this reason slippery elm is used as an ingredient in many herbal ointments and salves. Slippery elm tea can also be used as a gargle for sore throats.

Slippery elm bark is available in whole pieces, powdered, and shaped into tablets or lozenges. Do not harvest bark from wild or cultivated elm trees. American elms have been depleted by Dutch elm disease and should be protected from the widespread use of their bark. Fresh slippery elm bark is collected by wildcrafters and other naturalists who have obtained permits to do so. Slippery elm powder can be found in health-food stores and through wholesale and retail herb outlets.

Dried slippery elm powder must be stored in a dark, airtight jar, as it absorbs moisture quite easily. Keep the powder in a cupboard or closet, away from light and heat.

Valerian Root

— ◁◇▷ —

Valeriana officinalis

The valerian plant is a small perennial shrub growing to 4 feet in height, with tiny pointed leaves and pink, purple, or white flower clusters. Fresh valerian root is whitish-pink and odorless. The dried root is yellowish-gray in color and has a strong pungent smell.

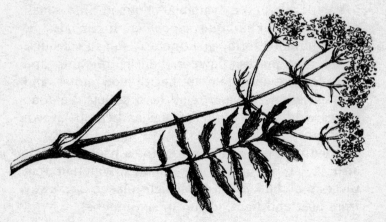

Valerian is native to Europe and has been naturalized in the United States. It grows in moist places, usually on the banks of streams or ditches. Only the root is used medicinally.

Valerian is a strong antispasmodic and tranquilizer and, as such, is a valuable and widely used herb. Its folk name, "all-heal," is a testament to its historic popularity. Because of the high content of volatile oils contained in valerian, it should not be boiled and drunk as a tea. Prepare it as a capsule, paste, or tincture instead. Powdered valerian root can be applied topically as a paste or ointment to relieve muscle cramps and spasms, headaches, and backaches. Taken internally as a tincture or tablet, valerian is effective against menstrual cramps, insomnia, nervousness, anxiety, and chronic stomach and intestinal upsets, especially when accompanied by nervous tension. Combined with other ingredients, valerian can regularize the hormone spikes of menopause. Valerian is also useful for calming people with heart conditions.

Valerian root is available chopped into small pieces and ground into a powder. It can also be found in tablet form, as a tincture, and in capsules. Dried root pieces, powder, tablets, tincture, and capsules are available in health-food stores and through wholesale and retail herb outlets. Valerian grows wild in the United States and can be grown easily in a pot or garden.

Dried valerian root powder stores well in a dark, airtight jar for up to four months. Valerian root pieces may be kept in an airtight plastic bag, away from heat and light, for up to six months.

Witch Hazel

—◄◊►—

Hamamelis virginiana

The small, gnarly hazel tree grows to a height of 15 feet and yields delicious, edible nuts. Hazel leaves are quite veiny and hairy, and the unusual hazel tree flowers only in autumn. The scaly, gray-brown outer bark, the shiny white inner bark, and the bitter-tasting leaves are all used medicinally.

Finding well water was an important survival skill for American settlers. Professional "water witches" cut the shoots of young hazel trees for use as divining rods when searching for underground water supplies. That's why this hazel is called "witch."

Witch hazel bark and leaves contain tannins, an active plant constituent useful for tanning hides. The effect of tannins on the body is astringent, and witch hazel extract dries and relieves the irritation of insect bites, cold sores, poison oak and ivy, and sunburn. A witch hazel sitz bath relieves the discomfort of hemorrhoids, reduces the pain and swelling of bruises, and restores tired feet. Applied as a wash, witch hazel reduces the swelling of varicose veins and relieves eye strain. A tea made from the bark and leaves is an excellent diarrhea remedy. Witch hazel extract is a beneficial ingredient in hair rinses and facial toners, as it dissolves oils produced by the skin and scalp.

Witch hazel is a common commercial extract found in pharmacies and grocery stores. Unfortunately, the tannins contained in the bark and leaves are lost in processing, and the resulting extract is not as astringent as even a simple decoction. For the purposes of this book, however, the extract still contains enough astringent properties to make it useful and expedient. Do not use the extract internally.

Less processed, though more expensive witch hazel extracts may be found in health-food stores, bath shops, and through wholesale and retail herb outlets. Store witch hazel extract in a tightly lidded jar in the medicine chest or linen closet.

Part 2

—◦⊳◦—

Symptoms and Recipes

The following section covers forty-two of the most common women's symptoms, their descriptions and causes, and their accompanying Cure Kit recipes.

A symptom is a sign or indication of something, usually of a particular physical disorder or of an abnormal emotional state of being. For total healing to occur, the entire system, the root causes as well as the symptoms, must be addressed. The herbal remedies included in the following section provide gentle relief from symptomatic discomfort and give you time and peace of mind to decide which healing methods and lifestyle changes will promote and maintain your overall health. However, the ideas, procedures, and suggestions in this book are intended to supplement, not replace, the medical advice of trained professionals. Consult your health-care practitioner if you decide to use herbal remedies for any condition that may require diagnosis or medical attention.

Each recipe in this section is a step-by-step preparation guide and includes symptom descriptions, information on probable causes, dosage recommendations, and expected results. Cross-referencing between recipes is provided if, in my opinion, a symptom responds best to a combination of remedies. Some of the recipes end with a discussion of when to see the doctor and include descriptions of symptoms too serious for self-diagnosis and healing. If one or more of these descriptions is applicable to you, I recommend the continued use of herbs for symptom relief and a consultation with a healing professional to decide the appropriate treatment for underlying disorders.

The following recipes are the results of my own independent research, of my training received through accredited herbal schools, and of experimental work I have performed with numerous teacher-practitioners. I have tested and retested each one for its simplicity, effectiveness, and safety, not only independently but also in conjunction with the many students I have taught over the years. The results achieved by using these recipes can range from fair to fantastic, but none of them will harm you. As long as you follow the guidelines I offer, they are perfectly safe. Your use of the fascinating and rewarding healing herbs is limited only by your imagination and creativity, combined with a healthy respect for following directions. As you perform your kitchen-cosmetic and medicinal rituals, I hope you experience, as I so often have, the feeling of pride, accomplishment, and simple wonder at producing your very own herbal cure.

Acne 🐝

Skin-Food Acne Remedy

———— ◄○► ————

Your skin sprouts pimples for many reasons, most of which we women have been intimately acquainted with since teenagerhood. Stress, smoking, diet, and hormones are all contributors, but the main cause, believe it or not, is dry skin. When your skin is dry and undernourished, facial pores produce too much oil, resulting in pimples.

Your skin is your body's largest organ, responsible for holding you together, eliminating wastes, and assimilating oxygen and moisture. Show some respect and feed your face with the following recipe.

> INGREDIENTS:
> ¼ cup almonds
> 1 cup ground oats
> ¼ cup cosmetic clay
> 1 tablespoon slippery elm powder
> 2 drops lavender oil
> 2 drops peppermint oil

With a food grinder, grind separately the almonds

and oats. Put the ground herbs in a metal bowl, add the cosmetic clay and the slippery elm powder, and sift the mixture with your fingers to combine. Stir in the lavender and peppermint oil with a metal spoon until the oils are completely absorbed. Combine one tablespoon of this dry-skin food mixture with any one of the following, one tablespoon at a time, until slightly moistened: yogurt, buttermilk, rose water, or plain water. Use this mixture as a scrub on a daily basis or mix it into a thicker paste for a weekly face mask. If you prefer a very thick paste, similar to a mud mask, increase the amount of dry ingredients and combine with mashed avocado, beaten egg, or honey.

APPLICATION: Use the facial scrub every morning. Massage vigorously over your face and neck, then rinse with warm water and pat dry. After rinsing, tone your skin with rose water or the Herbal Toner for Oily Skin (page 113). Finish by applying a cosmetic-grade sun block or a light daytime cream. Apply the Radiant Rose Moisture Cream (page 79) every night for round-the-clock moisturizing.

You can prepare and combine up to a pound of the dry Skin-Food Acne Remedy ingredients (including the lavender and peppermint oils) in advance. Store the dry mixture in an airtight, labeled plastic bag away from moisture, light, and heat. Discard the mixture after six months.

Anemia 🎀

Iron Woman Cocktail

————— ◄◦► —————

If you love to burn the candle at both ends, with cooking or even eating the last thing on your mind, be on the lookout for anemia. Fatigue, irritability, restlessness, and an inability to concentrate are the usual symptoms. Most women think about anemia only during pregnancy, but this condition is also caused by poor diet, stress, heavy periods, or loss of blood due to an accident or surgery.

Women used to get their iron the old-fashioned way, by cooking in cast-iron frying pans and pots. If, however, you would rather pump iron than cook with it, try the following delicious cocktail.

INGREDIENTS:
1 tablespoon black cherry extract
1 12-ounce glass of sparkling mineral water

Combine the extract with the mineral water in a tall glass. Stir thoroughly. You may sweeten the cocktail with honey or maple syrup or jazz it up with a wedge of lemon, lime, or orange.

APPLICATION: Drink the cocktail twice a day until your energy level gets up to where it should be. You will have good results immediately, as this form of organic iron is easily assimilated. If you are on the go and don't have time to mix the cocktail, bring a small bottle of the syrup with you and take a tablespoon neat twice a day until results are achieved. Wait until after eating to take the syrup by the spoonful or your blood sugar will go sky-high. Though it may seem like more is better with this harmless cocktail, don't exceed the recommended dosage, or digestive upset could result.

If you premix the cocktail in large amounts, store it in a ceramic or glass container and keep it chilled for up to a week. The plain syrup does not need to be refrigerated.

NOTE: Acute anemia is a serious condition and requires a physician's care. Symptoms of acute anemia include heart palpitations, breathlessness, facial pallor, insomnia, and chronic weakness. If you are experiencing any of these symptoms, consult a physician immediately.

Arthritis 🦋

Arthritis Ginger Pack

——— ◁◦▷ ———

Most of us have a "spot" on our bodies (mine is my right shoulder) where we hold tension. When muscle groups surrounding and connected to a joint become chronically tense and inflexible, painful arthritis-like inflammation results. Tight muscles are caused by injury, emotions, heredity, age, diet, or a combination of several of the above. Other common arthritis targets are knuckles, wrists, lower back, knees, and hips.

The following ginger pack helps relieve muscle tension and will return flexibility and fluidity of movement to your particular "spot."

> INGREDIENTS:
> ¼ cup powdered ginger root
> 2 tablespoons powdered cosmetic clay
> 20 drops peppermint oil
> 15 drops lavender oil
> hot water

Put the powdered ginger root and the cosmetic clay in a metal bowl and stir until thoroughly combined.

Add the oils of peppermint and lavender. Stir the mixture with a metal spoon until the oils have been absorbed. Add the hot water by the tablespoonful until a spreadable paste is formed.

APPLICATION: Spread a half-inch-thick layer of the warm mud pack onto the skin wherever you experience pain. Cover the pack with plastic wrap and a towel. If applying the pack to a joint, such as your knee, elbow, or finger, secure the pack with plastic wrap and a Band-Aid or Ace bandage. Keep the pack on for approximately forty-five minutes or until you feel your skin tingling and tightening beneath the herbs. Wash the compress off with very warm water, directing a strong flow to the area from a shower massager or nozzle, and finish with cold water. After the compress is washed away, massage the area with the Backache Balm (page 57) for continued pain relief.

You may mix large quantities of the dry ingredients and oils included in the Arthritis Ginger Pack ahead of time, and add hot water to a portion each time you wish to apply it. Keep the dry mixture for up to four months in a tightly lidded jar, away from moisture, heat, and light.

NOTE: If your arthritis or joint pain becomes severe, work with a qualified masseuse, chiropractor, physical therapist, or orthopedist to obtain further pain relief.

Backaches 🦋

Backache Balm

———— ◄◦► ————

Backaches range in severity from infrequent and mild to chronic and intolerable. Backache is the number-one reason for seeking a doctor's advice in this country, and there seem to be as many treatments for backache as there are causes. Improper lifting techniques, sitting too much, pregnancy, PMS, accidents, menopause, lack of exercise, and a host of other reasons too numerous to describe can tie your back in knots and leave you moaning on the couch.

A whirl in a Jacuzzi, followed by a Backache Balm rub, is my personal regimen for backache. Apply the balm yourself, if you must, but an extra set of caring hands provides complete relaxation.

INGREDIENTS:
1 cup olive oil
2 tablespoons grated fresh ginger root
1 tablespoon dried comfrey root pieces
2 tablespoons dried valerian root pieces
20 drops lavender oil
20 drops rosemary oil

40 drops peppermint oil
¼ cup grated beeswax

Combine the olive oil, grated ginger root, comfrey root pieces, and valerian root pieces in a slow-cooking pot set at low, or place the oil and herbs in a covered ovenproof dish and bake in the oven at a very low heat (200° F), for three to four hours. When the mixture is cured, strain out the herbs and discard. The oil will be dark brown, with a somewhat unpleasant, musty smell. Add the oils of lavender and rosemary and stir the mixture with a metal spoon. Return the oil to a heavy frying pan and add the beeswax. Gently heat the mixture until the beeswax is completely melted. Pour the hot ointment into a labeled glass jar and allow it to cool to room temperature. The opaque, dark-green ointment will solidify as it cools. Store the ointment away from heat and light and discard it after six months.

APPLICATION: Rub approximately two teaspoonfuls of the ointment into your back whenever you experience pain. Use more to cover larger areas.

NOTE: If you have frequent backaches, it could be because of misalignment of spinal vertebrae or an organic disorder. Consult with a chiropractor, physical therapist, osteopath, or physician for further advice.

Bladder Infections ❧

Barley Water Brew

——— ◄◦► ———

Women's urethras are approximately 1 inch long, and for this reason, your bladder has little protection from the outside world. Your inside plumbing often provides a stairway for bacteria hanging about in your panties, the local swimming pool, the public restroom, and so on. Excessive caffeine and alcohol intake, stress, poor diet, athletic sex, or the late stages of pregnancy can also irritate and inflame your bladder.

Although urinating is painful when you have a bladder infection or irritation, peeing a lot is the best way to get rid of it. The following brew will have you doing just that, with pain relief sure to follow.

INGREDIENTS:
½ cup pearled barley
1 quart water
1 teaspoon ginger root powder
1 tablespoon echinacea root powder
1 tablespoon goldenseal root powder
2 drops lavender oil

Combine the barley and water in a large covered pot, bring to a boil, and simmer for forty minutes. Strain the mixture, reserving the cooked barley for breakfast or as a thickener in soup. Return the barley water to the pot and add the ginger, echinacea, and goldenseal. Bring the mixture to a boil, and simmer for twenty minutes. Using a fine-mesh sieve, strain out and discard all the herb solids. Return the brew to a metal bowl and allow it to cool to a tepid temperature. Add the lavender oil and stir the mixture with a metal spoon. The brew will be milky and opaque, with a mild bitter smell.

APPLICATION: Drink one cup of brew three times a day. You may not like the taste of the tea, so add lemon juice and honey, or have an organic, unsweetened cranberry juice chaser on hand. Refrigerate the brew between servings. Discard any unused brew within two days. Consult with a physician if your symptoms persist after two days of treatment.

NOTE: Daily doses of the Echinacea and Goldenseal Sinus Tincture (see page 115), taken along with the Barley Water Brew, gives you extra infection-fighting power.

Breast Tenderness ❧

Tender Breast Massage Oil

——— ◄○► ———

When your breasts ache, every movement reminds you of their presence, not merely as part of your figure, but as part of your physical self. Pregnancy, premenstrual syndrome, sexual excitation, lactation, and hormone spikes during menopause all cause aching breasts. If you are the active type, breast tenderness is especially aggravating, in spite of your extra-support, cantilevered jog-bra.

The following massage oil is pleasant to use and will help relieve your aching breasts.

INGREDIENTS:
2 cups olive oil
1 ounce dried plantain leaves
1/2 ounce fresh rosemary leaves
10 drops peppermint oil
15 drops rosemary oil
15 drops lavender oil

Combine the plantain and rosemary leaves with the olive oil in a ceramic bowl. Stir the mixture with a wooden spoon until combined and let it rest for five minutes. Put the mixture in a slow-cooking pot set at low, or place the oil and herbs in a covered ovenproof dish and bake in the oven at a very low heat (200° F) for three to four hours. When the mixture is cured, strain out the herbs and discard. The oil should be dark green, with an earthy, woody fragrance. Add the oils of peppermint, lavender, and rosemary and stir the mixture with a metal spoon. Store the oil at room temperature in a labeled, lidded jar or plastic container for up to six months.

APPLICATION: Apply the warmed oil generously to your breasts. Gently rub in a circular motion, as though you were giving yourself a breast examination. Pay special attention to the sides of your breasts and your underarm area, where lymph nodes are susceptible to painful swelling. Use witch hazel solution or rose water to remove the oil and allow your breasts to air dry before dressing.

NOTE: If the soreness is severe or does not improve after three days of treatment, consult a physician. If you are a nursing mother and your breasts harden or turn red, or if you develop a fever, consult a physician. All women should consult a physician if new or unfamiliar lumps are discovered during a breast self-examination.

Burns (minor) ℘

Plantain Burn Poultice

———◄◦►———

Cooking is the primary cause of minor burns, with sunburns and small electrical shocks running a close second and third. When burns penetrate too deeply, painful, unsightly blisters develop, and the healing process is prolonged. Applying a cold pack to a minor, painful burn keeps the heat of the burn from penetrating to deeper levels of your skin.

The following poultice is an effective painkiller and skin regenerator. If you want to gourmandize without getting your fingers burned, keep some of the dried plantain in a jar near your stove.

INGREDIENTS:
3 tablespoons dried plantain leaves
juice from ½ lemon
4 ice cubes

Combine the plantain leaves, lemon juice, and ice cubes in a blender or food grinder. Whiz until the ice is crushed and the mixture resembles wet chopped grass. Let the poultice sit for two minutes, until the plantain swells and absorbs the ice-cold water and lemon juice. The mixture should be cold, dark green in color, and smell like lemony mown grass.

APPLICATION: Pat a small amount onto the burn area. If you have burned a small area on your finger or hand and wish to keep working, secure the poultice with a Band-Aid and carry on. If you are using the poultice for sunburn on your shoulders or back, double or triple the amount of ingredients (depending on the size of the area you wish to cover) and lie on your stomach while a helper pats the poultice on. Allow the poultice to do its stuff for at least twenty minutes. You may premix the plantain and lemon juice and refrigerate it if you are cooking a feast for twenty or are planning an all-day, out-of-doors, sun-exposure extravaganza. Discard the poultice after each use.

NOTE: This poultice is good for minor burns only. Second-degree burns, marked by redness, swelling, and blistering, or third-degree burns, caused by severe electrical shock or direct contact with fire or scalding water, require prompt medical attention.

Cold Sores 🍀

Goldenseal Cold Sore Tincture

———— ◄○► ————

Cold sores are ugly, painful, and attention-getting, besides being slow to heal. They are caused by a viral infection, which, under ideal conditions, your immune system usually keeps under control. If, however, your immune resistance is compromised by stress, poor diet, or iron-poor blood, icky cold sores, often accompanied by an equally icky cold, break out. Your mouth, nose, and eyes are the most vulnerable areas.

The following tincture will disinfect and dry out the most stubborn cold sores.

> INGREDIENTS:
> 2 tablespoons goldenseal powder
> 1 cup witch hazel extract

Pour the witch hazel extract into a spotlessly clean, quart-size jar with a tight-fitting lid. Add the goldenseal powder, screw on the lid, and shake the jar vigorously for two minutes. Label the jar with the date and name of the tincture, put it in a dark closet, and shake the jar for two minutes each day for the next two weeks. After that time, decant the tincture by straining out the goldenseal powder through a sieve lined with fine-weave cheesecloth. Discard the herb and return the strained mixture to the labeled jar. Keep the finished tincture away from light and heat. Discard leftover tincture after one year and make a fresh batch if necessary.

APPLICATION: Use a cotton ball to dab the cold sore with the tincture every night before going to bed. Continue this treatment until the cold sore dries up. Discontinue treatment with the tincture after the sore has closed and has started to dry. At this point, speed the healing process by applying rose water to the sore every morning, followed by a small dab of Radiant Rose Moisture Cream (page 79). Continue with this treatment until the sore has completely disappeared. For cold sores inside the mouth, dip a cotton swab in the tincture and gently dab it on the sore every night before going to bed.

NOTE: If the cold sores keep recurring, focus your healing strategies on your immune system. Consult with a physician or herbal practitioner for further information.

Constipation ❧

Anticonstipation Breakfast

———— ◄◊► ————

Our bodies have many ways of telling us to slow down, and constipation is one of them. A proper bowel movement proceeds at what I call a contemplative pace. Women (such as myself) who have themselves, their partners, and their children to get out of the door each morning often forget to take time for their most basic needs, and I'm not talking about hair and makeup.

The Anticonstipation Breakfast is a step-by-step procedure designed to help you focus on your dietary needs. Its proper use will ensure many rewarding contemplative moments.

> INGREDIENTS
> ½ cup organic rolled oats
> 1 tablespoon black cherry extract
> 2 cups water
> 1 teaspoon slippery elm powder

Combine the oats and black cherry extract with the water in a covered pot and allow the mixture to soak overnight. In the morning, add the slippery elm bark, bring the mixture to a boil, and simmer for fifteen minutes or until it is completely cooked. The finished consistency will be quite thick. When the oats are ready, spoon out a serving and add sweetener, milk, or your favorite fruit juice to taste.

APPLICATION: Eat a portion of the Anticonstipation Breakfast each morning until your bowel movements are regular and easy to pass. If you drink coffee or tea in the morning, decrease the amount you drink by half, or start using decaf, as caffeine irritates the bowels and counters the bulking and soothing effect of the oats. If you usually skip breakfast, take the oats mixture with you to work in a thermos and substitute it for your mid-morning pastry. The above recipe yields two servings. You may prepare the oats in bulk by doubling or tripling the recipe. Keep the mixture refrigerated until ready for use. Discard leftovers after one week and prepare a fresh batch if necessary.

NOTE: Chronic constipation can be a symptom of more serious bowel disorders. If moving your bowels causes pain, or if you experience uncomfortable cramping or bloating, consult with an herbal practitioner or physician.

Coughs ❧

Pennyroyal and Rosemary Steam

———— ◄◦► ————

Coughs interrupt phone conversations, laughter, whispered asides, sleep, and other daily necessities. Besides feeling somewhat unsophisticated during a coughing spell, you may also feel headachy, feverish, stuffed up, or grouchy. Coughs are caused by allergies, smoking, colds, asthma, or reactions to such airborne substances as paint thinner fumes or smoke.

Steam is a tried-and-true remedy for opening and cleansing mucous-clogged bronchial passages, and is especially helpful when combined with antiseptic inhalants such as pennyroyal and rosemary. Try the following steam for relief from irritating coughs.

> INGREDIENTS:
> 2 ounces dried pennyroyal leaves
> 6 drops rosemary oil
> 2 quarts cold water

Put the water and the dried pennyroyal in a pot and use a metal spoon to combine. Cover the pot and bring the mixture to a boil. Simmer for five minutes, then take the pot off the heat. Add the oil of rosemary and stir the mixture with a metal spoon. Place the pot wherever it is comfortable for you to sit or stand.

APPLICATION: Drape a large bath towel over your head and shoulders to form a tent over the pot as you bend over to inhale the steam. The steam will make your face feel a little hot. If you feel uncomfortable, come up for a cooling breath of air. Inhale the steam for five minutes, then uncover your head and breathe as deeply as you can for two minutes. During the break, cover the pot so that the water stays hot and no steam escapes. Repeat the process at least three times within thirty minutes, then discard the water and herbs. This treatment is good for one use only. Repeat the process once each night until the coughing improves.

NOTE: If your cough persists or grows worse after one week of treatment, or if you feel feverish or fatigued, consult with a physician.

Cuts (minor) 🐝

Boo-boo Balm

———— ‹○› ————

Cuts and scrapes go with the territory for those who enjoy hang-gliding, jumping from airplanes, rock climbing, warp-speed mountain biking, and other daring activities. If you are the more sedentary type, enjoying things like gardening, cooking, or refinishing dressers, you are still running a boo-boo risk. Let's face it, even if your favorite activity is reading a romance novel, life can still be dangerous. You might get a paper cut turning the page.

The following balm will disinfect your boo-boo, reduce pain and swelling, and help your skin to regenerate.

INGREDIENTS:
1 cup olive oil
1 tablespoon dried comfrey root pieces
1 tablespoon slippery elm bark pieces
1 teaspoon echinacea root powder
1 teaspoon goldenseal root powder
1 tablespoon grated lemon peel
20 drops lavender oil
1/4 cup grated beeswax

Combine the olive oil, comfrey root pieces, slippery elm bark pieces, echinacea root powder, goldenseal root powder, and grated lemon peel in a slow-cooking pot set at low, or place the oil and herbs in a covered ovenproof dish and bake in the oven at a very low heat (200° F) for three to four hours. When the mixture is cured, strain out the herbs with a fine-mesh sieve and discard. The oil should be dark brown, with a pungent, earthy odor. Return the oil to a cast-iron frying pan and add the beeswax. Gently heat the mixture until the beeswax is completely melted. Remove the pan from the heat. With a metal spoon, stir in the oil of lavender and pour the hot mixture into a labeled glass jar. Allow the ointment to cool to room temperature. The opaque, dark-brown ointment will solidify as it cools. Store the jar of ointment away from heat and light and discard it after six months.

APPLICATION: Rub the ointment into your cut or scrape after cleansing.

NOTE: This balm is for minor cuts and scrapes only. If a wound is large or deep, stitches may be needed to close it. Deep puncture wounds require a tetanus shot if ten years has passed since your last immunization.

Dandruff ❧

Dandruff Hair Rinse

———— ◄○► ————

Dandruff causes discomfort to both your vanity and your pocketbook. It is caused by poor scalp circulation and is aggravated by poor diet, stress, and hormonal imbalances.

Our foremothers had many ways of keeping their crowning glory in good condition. Brushing the hair each night one hundred times with a boar-bristle brush to stimulate scalp circulation was one of their many secrets. If you have neither the patience nor the forearms for such a treatment, try the following rinse.

INGREDIENTS:
1 ounce dried rosemary leaves
1 quart cold water
10 drops lavender oil
5 drops peppermint oil
2 tablespoons commercial witch hazel extract

Immerse the rosemary leaves in the cold water, bring to a boil, and simmer gently for twenty minutes in a tightly covered pot. Place a cheesecloth-lined strainer in a large bowl and pour the hot rinse into it. After the liquid drains into the bowl, gather the corners of the cheesecloth and squeeze the remaining rinse out of the rosemary leaves. Discard the cheesecloth and leaves. The rinse should be greenish-gold in color and smell sharply of rosemary. After the rinse has cooled to room temperature, add the witch hazel tincture and the oils of lavender and peppermint. Stir the mixture with a metal spoon to combine. This recipe provides enough rinse for one application. You may double or triple the recipe and store the rinse in a clean, labeled jar with a tight-fitting lid for up to two weeks.

APPLICATION: Pour the rinse through your hair after washing with a mild shampoo. Vigorously massage the rinse into your hair and scalp. Catch the runoff in a bowl and repeat the procedure. Pour the rinse over your hair one final time and wrap your head in a thick towel to dry; then proceed with styling. Use the rinse each time you shampoo, or until your dandruff disappears.

Diarrhea 🦠

Runs Remedy

——◀◉▶——

This inconvenient malady can ruin the best-laid of plans. Diarrhea is usually caused by ingestion of tainted food or some other kind of intestinal upset, although certain emotional states can also get your bowels in an uproar. Shock or terror are powerful emotional evacuators, and even harmless little feelings like tension or indecisiveness can contribute to what was once called "the skitters."

If you find yourself in this lamentable condition, avoid cooked and raw green vegetables and acidic fruits. Applesauce and yogurt make a good antidiarrhea combination, along with the following tea.

INGREDIENTS:
½ cup pearled barley
1 teaspoon slippery elm powder
1 quart water
½ cup culinary rose water

Combine the barley, slippery elm powder, and water in a large covered pot, bring to a boil, and simmer for twenty minutes. Using a fine-mesh sieve, strain the mixture into a metal bowl and mash the herbs with a flat spoon to extract all of the moisture. Discard the cooked herbs. Allow the barley–slippery elm water to cool to a tepid temperature and add the rose water. Stir the mixture with a metal spoon to combine. The liquid will be milky and opaque, with a pleasant rose scent.

APPLICATION: Drink the Runs Remedy, five times a day, a half a cup at a time, until the diarrhea has abated. If you simply must go to work or elsewhere, bring the remedy with you in a thermos. Some thermos cups are premeasured; if yours isn't, eyeball an approximate half-cup each time you drink it.

NOTE: The physical cramping and discomfort of diarrhea can be relieved with the following belly rub oil. Combine six drops of lavender oil with two tablespoons of olive or almond oil. Starting on your right side just below your rib cage, massage the oil in a circular motion onto your abdomen until the pain is relieved.

Dry or Damaged Hair ❧

Hot Herbal Oil Treatment

———— ◄○► ————

Hair that is permed, hot-curled, colored, teased, or sunburned once too often will end up frizzy, dry, and limp. Each hair shaft needs moisture-laden cells lining it to reflect shine and add bounce and body to your do. The same things that dry out your skin also dry out your hair, including washing or shampooing with strong detergent shampoos, swimming in chlorinated pools, smoking, stress, and poor diet.

The baffling array of dry-hair products available in stores each claim an exclusive hair-healing formula. If you would rather not spend the better part of a day trying to decide which one to use, try my oldie-but-goodie dry-hair remedy.

INGREDIENTS:
2 cups olive oil
1 ounce comfrey root pieces
20 drops lavender oil
20 drops rosemary oil

Combine the comfrey root pieces with the olive oil

in a ceramic bowl. Stir the mixture with a wooden spoon and let it rest for five minutes. Put the mixture in a slow-cooking pot set at low, or place the oil and comfrey root pieces in a covered ovenproof dish and bake in the oven at a very low heat (200° F) for three to four hours. When the mixture is cured, strain out the herbs and discard. The oil should be dark brown in color, with a musty earth fragrance. Add the oils of lavender and rosemary and stir the mixture with a metal spoon. Store the oil at room temperature in a labeled, lidded glass jar for up to six months.

APPLICATION: Put a cotton towel in a large pot, add water to cover, and heat the water to a tepid temperature. While the water in the large pot is heating, place the glass jar containing the oil in a small pot of cold water. Warm the water until small bubbles form in the bottom of the pot. Remove the pot from the heat and pour a tablespoon of the warmed oil into your palm. Rub your hands together and vigorously massage the oil into your scalp and hair strands. Repeat the procedure until your hair is saturated from roots to ends. Cover your head with plastic wrap or a plastic shower cap. Wring out the hot towel and wrap it around your head. When the towel cools, dip it in the hot water, wring it out well, and rewrap your hair. Treat your hair for at least thirty minutes, then wash the oil out with a mild shampoo. Use the Hot Herbal Oil Treatment at least two times, once a week, to see results. You may also use it indefinitely as a once-a-week beauty treatment to keep your hair shining and healthy.

Dry Skin 🌹

Radiant Rose Moisture Cream

———— ◄◦► ————

Moist skin imparts a dewy, youthful look. Work that requires you to be outdoors, or activities like swimming, hiking, and skiing can give you a taut, leathery look, even if you wear sun block. Dry skin casualties include wrinkles, bags, sags, crow's-feet, and other facial fashion flaws. Smoking and stress also reduce the skin's moisture content.

Rose-petal complexions were once protected by hats, parasols, and milk baths. If you prefer a less complicated approach, try the following recipe.

INGREDIENTS:
1½ cups almond oil
½ ounce grated beeswax
⅔ cup distilled rose water
⅓ cup aloe vera gel

Combine the almond oil and the beeswax in a double boiler. Heat just enough to melt the beeswax into the almond oil. When the beeswax is completely melted and the mixture is clear, pour it into a glass measuring cup and let it cool to room temperature. The mixture will become cloudy as it cools. When the oil mixture is room temperature, put the rose water and aloe vera gel in a blender and mix on the highest speed. Slowly pour the cooled oil into the liquid ingredients as they blend. Turn off the blender when the mixture becomes thick and white (in approximately two minutes). The moisture cream will thicken further as it sets.

APPLICATION: This cream is for nighttime use only. After washing and toning your skin for the night, apply a small amount of moisture cream to your face and neck. Thoroughly blend the cream into your skin every night for maximum results.

Store the moisture cream at room temperature in a labeled, clean glass jar with a tight-fitting lid. Keep the moisture cream away from light and heat. Discard any unused cream after six months and mix up a fresh batch.

Eye Strain 🦋

Soothing Eye Strain Routine

—◄◦►—

Cramming for an exam, preparing a legal case, developing a software program, and other activities requiring intense visual concentration often result in eye strain. Less obvious causes include undiagnosed visual problems and incorrect or outdated eyeglass prescriptions. Unrelieved eye strain causes headaches, nausea, and general fatigue. Besides feeling miserable, you don't look your best, either, as tired eyes become bloodshot, puffy, or encircled with dark pouches.

Once you have had your eyes checked to eliminate the possibility of needing glasses or a different lens prescription, try the following soothing procedure.

INGREDIENTS:
1/4 cup commercial witch hazel tincture
1 cup boiled or distilled water
1/4 cup rose water
1/4 cup aloe vera gel
gauze pads
cotton balls

Put the water in a covered pot and warm to a tepid temperature. While the water is heating, combine the rose water and aloe vera gel in a blender. Transfer the aloe vera–rose water mixture to a small metal bowl and set it aside. Add the witch hazel tincture to the warmed water and stir the mixture with a metal spoon.

APPLICATION: Find a comfortable place to lie down and arrange all of your ingredients there. Soak the gauze pads in the witch hazel–water solution, gently wring out the excess, and apply the pads to your eyes. When the pads become cool, soak them again in the warm solution and reapply. Repeat this procedure for twenty minutes, then discard the solution. Next, use a cotton ball to apply the mixture of aloe vera gel and rose water to the area surrounding your eyes. Do not apply it to your eyelids or eye tissue. Let the mixture dry on your skin, then gently rinse the eye area with warm water. Your eyes should feel and look better. Repeat this procedure once a day or until eye strain is relieved. This formula is good for one application only.

NOTE: If your eyes are itchy, bloodshot, or tearing, or if you suffer from frequent headaches, consult with an allergist, ophthalmologist, or physician.

Foot Problems 🌢

Rosemary Foot Refresher

————— ◄◌► —————

Nothing can ruin your day more thoroughly than sore feet. Work that requires lots of walking or standing, and physical activities like hiking, running, and dancing can really get your dogs barking, especially if you've been wearing shoes for fashion rather than fit. Your overworked feet protect themselves by developing corns and callouses, which only result in more discomfort.

A good foot rub can bring relief for many of the above symptoms, but if no one is willing and available, here is a comforting foot-bath ritual.

> INGREDIENTS:
> 2 ounces fresh, finely chopped rosemary
> 1/4 cup almond oil
> 15 drops rosemary oil
> 15 drops lavender oil
> 2 gallons hot water
> 1 bottle commercial witch hazel extract

Find a comfortable place for a foot bath and arrange all your ingredients there. Combine the fresh, chopped rosemary and the almond oil in a small ceramic bowl. Mix with your fingers until it can form a ball in the palm of your hand. Set the mixture aside. Pour the hot water into a container large enough to hold both your feet. The water should be as hot as you can stand without risking a burn. Add the rosemary and lavender oil to the water and immerse your feet. Relax for a minute or two.

APPLICATION: Lift one foot out of the water and rest it across your knee. Gently scrub a palmful of the rosemary mixture onto your skin, letting the excess fall into the bathwater. Be sure to scrub your ankles as well as the toes, tops, and soles of your feet. When both your feet are done, immerse them in the water and relax. The chopped rosemary leaves will exude a delightful aroma as they float in the bath.

Relax with the foot bath for as long as you like. When your feet feel soothed and refreshed, dry them with a thick bath towel. Apply a few palmfuls of witch hazel to both feet, then put them up and allow them to air dry.

This foot bath is good for one use only.

Hair Loss 🍀

Hair-Loss Hair Oil

———— ◄○► ————

Men aren't the only people affected by hair loss. We women usually see our hair as just another accessory to be curled, colored, or cut, but older women, postpartum women, and women experiencing chemotherapy or some other powerful systemic change can lose this taken-for-granted accessory by the fistful. Progressive hair loss is emotionally devastating, as it changes your appearance in an uncontrolled way and prompts painful comments and questions from the indiscreet.

The following hair oil can slow or reverse the hair-loss process. More importantly, this procedure gives a woman a beautiful way to restore growth and health to both her hair and her spirit.

INGREDIENTS:
3 ounces olive oil
½ ounce rosemary oil
20 drops lavender oil

Combine the olive oil, the oil of rosemary, and the oil of lavender in a metal bowl. Stir with a metal spoon until the oils are completely combined. Pour the hair oil into a labeled glass jar with a tight-fitting lid. Store the jar in a cool place, away from heat and light. Discard any unused oil after six months.

APPLICATION: Before retiring for the night, place the glass jar containing the oil in a small pot of cold water. Warm the water until small bubbles form in the bottom of the pot. Remove the pot from the heat and pour a small amount of the warmed oil into your palm. Rub your hands together and gently massage the oil into your scalp and hair strands. Repeat the procedure until your hair is saturated, from roots to ends. Cover your head with plastic wrap or a plastic shower cap to keep the oil from staining your bed linen. In the morning, wash the oil out with mild castile or olive oil–based shampoo. Repeat this procedure every other night until results are achieved.

NOTE: Unexplained hair loss can be caused by alopecia, a skin disease that causes head hair, eyebrows, and eyelashes to fall out. If you are experiencing these symptoms, develop a treatment plan with a dermatologist or other physician.

Hangover 🐞

Ginger Rose Hangover Tonic

———— ◄◘► ————

Excessive consumption of alcohol irritates your stomach, liver, and kidneys and initiates the biological rebellion known as a hangover. Nausea, severe head- and muscle-aches, fatigue, and thirst are the usual symptoms. One way of avoiding a hangover, besides avoiding alcohol altogether, is to drink equal amounts of water and alcohol whenever you choose to imbibe.

Although getting out of bed after you finally wake up may feel like an unacceptable risk, make your painful way to the kitchen and brew a dose of this pleasant tea. It takes the edge off the morning after.

INGREDIENTS:
1 tablespoon finely chopped fresh ginger root
1 teaspoon grated lemon peel
2 cups water
$1/4$ cup culinary rose water
1 drop peppermint oil

Combine the ginger root, lemon peel, and water in a covered pot, bring to a boil, and simmer for ten minutes. Strain out the ginger and lemon peel pieces and discard them. Return the tea to a metal bowl and allow it to cool for ten minutes. Add the rose water and oil of peppermint and stir the mixture with a metal spoon. The tonic will be light yellow in color and smell pleasantly of ginger, rose, and peppermint. You may add lemon juice, honey, or maple syrup to taste.

APPLICATION: Drink half a cup of the tonic every two hours throughout the day to help control headache, nausea, and general lassitude. Drink plain water between doses, to flush your liver and kidneys and to relieve thirst. The tonic provides a delightful rose aftertaste that is probably far preferable to what you woke up with. Keep the brew at room temperature between servings and warm it to a comfortable drinking temperature for each use. Discard any unused brew when you feel better.

NOTE: The Headache Head Rub (page 91) may come in handy to help relieve your poor head.

Head Congestion 🐝

Head Congestion Bath

———— ◁◇▷ ————

Though facials are specific for head congestion, I have found herbal baths a pleasant alternative to hanging out over a hot pot. If your head is clogged because of a cold or flu, an herbal bath warms you and increases your immune resistance as it clears your clogged head. A hot bath enhanced by herbal oils and ingredients is also beneficial in the case of hay fever, sinusitis, and other allergy complaints.

Bathing, though much more time-consuming than showering, is a wonderful way to retreat and re-group. The following bath, which will clear your head and refresh your body, is worth the time it takes.

INGREDIENTS:
1/4 cup grated fresh ginger root pieces
1 ounce dried pennyroyal leaves
2 quarts water
20 drops peppermint oil
20 drops rosemary oil

Combine the fresh ginger root pieces and dried pennyroyal leaves with the water in a covered pot, bring to a boil, and simmer slowly for twenty minutes. Strain out and discard the herbs. Pour this tea and the oils of peppermint and rosemary into the bathtub while running the bath to ensure it will be well combined with the bathwater. Run the bath as hot as your usual bath temperature. Just before entering the bath, stir the water with your hand until the tea and oils are well combined. The bathwater will be a light greenish-brown, with a refreshing ginger-camphor-mint smell.

APPLICATION: Soak in the bath for twenty minutes or longer. Inhale deeply through your nose and mouth to enhance the decongestant and anti-inflammatory effects of the herbs. Don't worry if the oils in the bath make your skin tingle slightly, just enjoy the sensation. Take the bath once each day until your head congestion is relieved. Use the bath in the late afternoon after returning from work or your daytime activities, but not just before bed, as it is slightly stimulating.

Headaches 🦋

Headache Head Rub

———— ◄◉► ————

Of all the miserable ills flesh is heir to, headaches
have to be the worst. The many causes and varieties
of headache, including migraine, allergic reaction,
tension, and hangover, all have one symptom in
common: pain. The fact that headaches, for the
most part, are invisible makes matters worse.
Though your suffering should be obvious to those
who really care, getting some sympathy may require
dramatic attention-getting displays, including lying
full-length on the couch and groaning or holding
your head in your hands while pacing around your
living room.

When you get tired of such displays, or you find
yourself deserted by friends and family, use the following helpful rub.

INGREDIENTS:
1/4 cup almond oil
20 drops rosemary oil
20 drops lavender oil
30 drops peppermint oil

Combine the almond oil and the oils of rosemary, lavender, and peppermint in a metal bowl. Gently stir the mixture with a metal spoon until the oils are thoroughly combined. Pour the headache oil into a labeled glass jar with a tight-fitting lid; it may be stored in a cool place, away from light and heat, for up to six months.

APPLICATION: Massage the oil onto the forehead and temples with gentle, rhythmic movements. Apply a small amount inside each nostril so that the vapors may be inhaled. This treatment usually brings quick relief, but if the headache persists, rub the oil vigorously into the back of your neck, at the base of your skull. You may obtain additional relief by rubbing the oil into the web of flesh between your thumb and forefinger, where a headache-relieving acupressure point is located. Because rubbing this point stimulates the metabolism, this procedure is not recommended for pregnant women.

NOTE: Ten drops of Valerian Root Insomnia Tincture (page 97) in an eight-ounce glass of hot water tastes terrible but helps relieve headaches. Use this tea along with the Headache Head Rub for a more thorough treatment, but keep in mind that the tea may cause drowsiness.

Headaches can be a symptom of underlying physiological disorders or postural abnormalities. Consult with a holistic practitioner, chiropractor, or physician if you suffer from persistent headaches.

Hemorrhoids 🦋

Hot Seat Hemorrhoid Ointment

———— ◅◦► ————

Hemorrhoids are congested, swollen veins and capillaries in the anal area. Many women endure the itching and pain of hemorrhoids during the late stages of pregnancy and the period immediately following childbirth, and they are comforted by knowing their condition is temporary. Hemorrhoids are chronic for other women, and can become risky business if they start to bleed (see note below). Causes of chronic hemorrhoids include constipation, sedentary lifestyle, straining during bowel movements, frequent use of laxatives, and emotional tension.

Fortunately, relief from the immediate discomfort of hemorrhoids is provided by the following ointment recipe.

INGREDIENTS:
1 cup olive oil
2 tablespoons dried plantain
1 tablespoon dried comfrey root pieces
1 tablespoon powdered goldenseal root
¼ cup grated beeswax

Combine the olive oil, dried plantain, comfrey root pieces, and powdered goldenseal root in a slow-cooking pot set at low, or place the oil and herbs in a covered ovenproof dish and bake in the oven at a very low heat (200° F) for three to four hours. When the mixture is cured, strain out and discard the herbs. The oil should be dark brown, with a grassy earth smell. Return the oil to a cast-iron frying pan and add the beeswax. Gently heat the mixture until the beeswax is completely melted. Pour the hot ointment into a labeled glass jar and allow it to cool to room temperature. The opaque, dark brown ointment solidifies as it cools.

APPLICATION: Keep the oil in the refrigerator at all times. Apply the cold oil directly to the anal area. It will be a rude shock to feel something cold in such a sensitive area, but cold constricts swollen veins and reduces discomfort. To remove the oil, gently wipe the area with a cotton ball soaked in witch hazel extract. Keep the witch hazel extract refrigerated also, if you can stand it.

NOTE: Severe hemorrhoids sometimes rupture and bleed, especially during a bowel movement. Bleeding in the anal area can result in infection and the formation of scar tissue. If you are bleeding from the anal area, consult with a physician.

Hot Flashes 🍀

Hot Flash Helper

———— ◄◦► ————

A hot flash is barely noticed by some women, while for others it's as if they just stepped in front of a blast furnace. A hot flash starts as a sudden rush of heat to the head and face and rapidly spreads to the rest of the body. The secondary effects of a hot flash include breaking out in a free sweat, flushing beet-red, or experiencing a rapid rise in heartbeat. Some women feel dizzy or tired after the hot flash subsides.

If you've been plagued by some or all of these symptoms, try the following tincture.

> INGREDIENTS:
> 2 cups high-quality vodka
> 1 tablespoon dong quai root pieces
> 1 tablespoon valerian root pieces
> 2 tablespoons oats
> 1 teaspoon goldenseal root powder

Pour the vodka into a spotlessly clean, quart-size jar with a tight-fitting lid. Add the remaining ingredients in the order given. Screw on the lid and shake the jar vigorously for two minutes. Label the jar with the date and name of the tincture, put it in a dark closet, and shake the jar for two minutes each day for the next two weeks. After that time, decant the tincture by straining out the herbs through fine-weave cheesecloth. Discard the herbs and return the strained mixture to the labeled jar. Keep the finished tincture away from light and heat. Discard leftover tincture after one year and make a fresh batch if necessary.

APPLICATION: Give yourself five drops under the tongue each time you feel a hot flash starting. Do not do this more than five times a day. If you are on the go, keep a one-ounce dropper bottle of tincture in your purse or cosmetic case.

NOTE: A splash of scented water on the face and wrists can cool you during a hot flash. Fill a two-ounce spray bottle with rose water, add one drop of peppermint oil, and shake vigorously to combine. Spray yourself generously whenever you feel the heat start to rise. Carry this spray along with the tincture and use them in combination.

Insomnia ❧

Valerian Root Insomnia Tincture

——— ◄◦► ———

The most common form of insomnia is an inability to relax, or "drop off," into sleep, usually caused by impending nerve-wracking situations, such as job interviews, weddings, or production deadlines. These occasional events cause your nervous system to remain on "yellow alert" and make falling asleep difficult. The other form of insomnia, less common but more insidious, is caused by unrelieved stress or depression. Symptoms include waking in the wee hours with nervous thoughts chasing each other around in your hyperactive brain, resulting in increased irritability and jumpiness during the day.

The following recipe soothes and rejuvenates your jangled nerves, and allows you to get some much-needed rest.

INGREDIENTS:
2 cups high-quality vodka
2 tablespoons valerian root pieces
2 tablespoons oats

Pour the vodka into a spotlessly clean quart-size jar

with a tight-fitting lid. Add the remaining ingredients in the order given. Screw on the lid and shake the jar vigorously for two minutes. Label the jar with the date and name of the tincture, put it in a dark closet, and shake the jar for two minutes each day for the next two weeks. Decant the tincture by straining out the herbs through fine-weave cheesecloth. Discard the herbs and return the strained mixture to the labeled jar. Keep the finished tincture away from light and heat. Discard leftover tincture after one year and make a fresh batch if necessary.

APPLICATION: Give yourself ten to fifteen drops under the tongue at night when you can't sleep. This tincture tastes nasty, so keep a warmed drink of milk or water on hand for a quick chaser. Allow at least an hour to pass before repeating the procedure. Do not take three doses in one night or you will have difficulty waking up the next day.

NOTE: Place one drop of lavender oil and one drop of peppermint oil on a tissue or hanky. Allow the oils to spread and dry slightly. Put the scented tissue or hanky inside your pillowcase and inhale the calming essences as you rest. Sweet dreams.

Liver Spots ❧

Delightful Skin-Whitening Paste

———— ◄◦► ————

Liver spots love to congregate on your face and hands, where all the world can easily see them. Also called age spots—another great name—they are caused by overexposure to the sun's harmful rays. A sprinkling of freckles was once considered unladylike, as it betrayed the wearer's tomboyish love of the outdoors. Ladies were supposed to stay hidden inside, serving tea or something. Obviously, times have changed and freckles are in, but liver spots will probably never be considered fashionable.

The following paste recipe is fun to make and will whiten and soften your skin.

INGREDIENTS:
1 cup cosmetic rose water
1 cup lemon juice
$\frac{1}{2}$ cup finely ground almonds
$\frac{1}{2}$ cup finely ground oats

Put the rose water and lemon juice in a metal bowl and stir with a metal spoon to combine. Pour off one cup of the rose water–lemon juice mixture and set aside. Add the ground almonds and ground oats to the remaining liquids. Stir the mixture vigorously until thickened and combined. If the paste becomes too thick, add buttermilk, yogurt, or plain milk, a tablespoon at a time, to thin the mixture to a spreadable consistency.

APPLICATION: Pat the paste onto your face, neck, and shoulders and leave it there to dry. While the face mask is drying, apply the paste to your hands, wrists, or anywhere else on your body, as needed. Allow the paste to dry completely before removing. Remove the paste by rinsing with warm water at the sink, or if necessary, in a warm bath. After removing the paste, rinse the skin with the mixture of plain rose water and lemon juice and allow it to air dry. Repeat this procedure once a day until the liver spots have started to fade. You may grind the dry ingredients in volume ahead of time and store them for up to one month in a clean glass jar with a tight-fitting lid. Prepare fresh liquid ingredients each time you prepare the paste, discarding any leftovers after one day.

NOTE: This is a slow process and may take many repetitions. Don't be alarmed if the spots seem to darken at first. The layers of skin are peeling away, heightening the contrast between light and dark. When used correctly and consistently, this recipe can fade or erase liver spots; but it is not guaranteed to completely erase all liver spots. Consult a dermatologist if any spot or blemish on your body starts to inexplicably darken, harden, or change its shape.

Menstrual Cramping ❧

Pennyroyal Belly Rub

———— ◅◦▻ ————

Menstrual cramping, which can range from mild to extremely painful, is a common condition among women of childbearing age. You may experience cramps as a dull, achy, heavy feeling in your lower abdomen and back, or as a spasmodic pain centered only in your pelvis. Your uterus is a powerful muscle that contracts in response to menstrual hormonal stimulation. Like any other muscle in your body, it will respond to a soothing rub.

The following belly massage oil recipe contains pennyroyal, a popular and very effective herb.

INGREDIENTS:
1 cup almond oil
½ ounce dried pennyroyal leaves

Combine the pennyroyal leaves with the almond oil in a ceramic bowl. Stir the mixture vigorously with a wooden spoon and let it rest for five minutes. Put the mixture in a slow-cooking pot set at low, or place the oil and pennyroyal leaves in a covered, ovenproof dish and bake in the oven at a very low heat (200° F) for three to four hours. When the mixture is cured, strain out and discard the pennyroyal leaves. The oil should be pale yellow, with a strong camphor-mint fragrance. Store the oil at room temperature in a labeled, lidded jar for up to six months.

APPLICATION: Place the glass jar containing the oil in a small pot of cold water. Warm the water until small bubbles form in the bottom of the pot. Remove the pot from the heat and pour a tablespoonful of the warmed oil into your palm. Apply the warmed oil sparingly to your lower abdomen and back whenever you experience menstrual cramping. Use the oil right after a bath, and gently rub it into the skin until it is absorbed. Relief is usually immediate. After you have finished your massage, rest on a couch or bed with your feet up, supporting your back with pillows. If you are on the go, keep a tightly lidded one-ounce jar of the oil with you in your purse and apply small amounts as needed.

NOTE: If your menstrual cramping is severe or prolonged, it may be a secondary effect resulting from some other disorder. Consult with a physician for correct diagnosis and treatment.

Morning Sickness 🦋

Preggers Tea

———— ◆ ————

As many women know, morning sickness isn't necessarily confined to morning, nor is food the only thing that makes you feel sick. Sometimes a whiff of bus exhaust is enough to send you running for a bathroom. Your senses of smell and taste are heightened during pregnancy, which, depending on whether you are in a garden or near the city dump, can be a mixed blessing.

Though many remedies exist for nauseated stomachs, not all of them are suitable for pregnant women. The following recipe is safe, simple, and effective, even for those days when nothing seems to stay down.

INGREDIENTS:
1 quart water
1 tablespoon oats
2 tablespoons pearled barley
1 teaspoon slippery elm bark powder
1 teaspoon grated fresh ginger root
1 drop peppermint oil

103

Combine the oats, pearled barley, slippery elm bark powder, and ginger root in a metal bowl. Stir with a metal spoon until combined. Add the mixture to the water and simmer gently for twenty minutes in a tightly covered pot. Place a strainer in a large bowl and pour the tea into it. After the liquid drains into the bowl, lift the strainer up and, with a wooden spoon, mash the mixture and squeeze any remaining tea out of the gruel. Discard the gruel.

Allow the mixture to cool to drinking temperature. Add the peppermint oil and stir with a metal spoon. The tea will smell and taste mildly of ginger, and it will be slightly opaque. You may add honey or maple syrup to taste. Refrigerate any unused portion of the tea. Discard it after one week.

APPLICATION: Drink half a cup of the warmed tea upon rising and before going to bed every day. Fill a small thermos with the mixture and sip it throughout the day whenever you feel the need. Some women feel sick only after eating; if this is you, drink a few sips immediately before and after each meal to soothe your stomach and help food stay down.

Muscle Tension 🐝

Muscle Tension Bath

———◄◊►———

Even if your body is required to do nothing more than carry your brain around, you can still get tense muscles, especially in your lower back, shoulders, or neck. Muscles bunch and tighten to protect themselves from overexertion caused by exercise, poor posture, or nerves. Whatever is causing your muscles to tighten, there is nothing like a hot bath to loosen them up. Heat fills the muscles, tendons, and ligaments with blood, and helps them relax.

Showers, or shower-baths as they were once called, were invented to massage the muscles and invigorate the skin. Follow your hot bath with a quick cold shower for maximum relaxation.

INGREDIENTS:
cotton bath bag
2 tablespoons grated fresh ginger root
1 ounce fresh rosemary
20 drops rosemary oil
20 drops lavender oil
1 cup rose water

Create a cotton bath bag by cutting a 1-foot-square piece of fine-weave cheesecloth. Place the fresh, grated ginger root and fresh rosemary in the middle. Gather two of the four corners and tie them together. Gather the remaining two corners and tie them also. With a piece of string, ribbon, or extra cheesecloth, tie the bath bag to the spigot of your bathtub and allow hot bathwater to run through it as you draw your bath. When your bath is full, take the bath bag from the spigot and allow it to float in the bathwater. Add the rose water and rosemary and lavender oil and swirl the bathwater with your hand to combine. The bathwater will be pale yellow in color and should smell like a flowering herb garden.

APPLICATION: Soak in the tub for at least twenty minutes. Take the bath bag and vigorously rub it onto your skin wherever your muscles are tight and tense. Your skin will tingle pleasantly wherever you rub the bag. When you have finished your rub, lie back and relax as completely as you can for the remainder of your bath.

Nausea 🙌

Herbal Bitters for Nausea

——— ◄◦► ———

Your stomach is a twenty-four-hour barometer, carefully charting and weighing your emotional and physical state. Along with its usual task of telling you when you are hungry, your stomach reacts to motions, sights, smells, emotional states, and even repetitive sounds. You already know about motion sickness if you've ever tossed your cookies over the side of a boat or out the window of a car. Think also of when your stomach has butterflies or shrinks to the size of a walnut because of fear, emotional trauma, or shock.

Other, more mundane, reasons for a rebellious stomach include conspicuous consumption of alcohol, eating spoiled or excessively rich food, and flu. To keep your stomach under control, try the following recipe of herbal bitters.

INGREDIENTS:
2 cups high-quality vodka
2 tablespoons grated fresh ginger root pieces
1 teaspoon powdered goldenseal root
1 tablespoon dried dong quai root pieces
1 tablespoon dried plantain
5 drops peppermint oil

Pour the vodka into a spotlessly clean quart-size jar with a tight-fitting lid. Add the remaining ingredients in the order given. Screw on the lid and shake the jar vigorously for two minutes. Label the jar with the date and name of the tincture, put it in a dark closet, and shake the jar for two minutes each day for the next two weeks. Decant the tincture by straining out the herbs through fine-weave cheesecloth. Discard the herbs and return the strained mixture to the labeled jar. Keep the finished tincture away from light and heat. Discard leftover tincture after one year and make a fresh batch if necessary.

APPLICATION: Put ten drops of the tincture in an eight-ounce mug of hot water whenever you feel nauseated. Stir to combine and drink the contents of the mug as quickly as you can. Repeat this procedure every hour until you feel better. Prepare the tea in advance and put it in a thermos if you're obliged to travel by air, sea, or land.

NOTE: Do not use this remedy for morning sickness. Refer to Preggers Tea (page 103). If nausea persists for more than two days or occurs frequently, consult with a holistic practitioner or physician.

Nervous Tension 🍂

Nervous Tension Massage Oil

——— ◁◦▷ ———

Moving from one house to another, entertaining in-laws, or making that big sale are all temporary tension builders. Caring for young children, working too hard, relationship problems, or a dreadful combination of all three can cause long-term tension, leaving you unable to unwind even in the most relaxing circumstances. When nervous tension becomes a state of mind and body, a host of physical and emotional ailments ensue, including headaches, irritability, short temper, jumpiness, and insomnia.

Feeling stuck forever in your own personal obstacle course starts the nervous-tension cycle. Break the pattern and get things in perspective with a full-body massage using the following massage-oil recipe.

INGREDIENTS:
1 cup almond oil
2 tablespoons finely grated lemon peel
2 tablespoons chopped fresh rosemary leaves
20 drops lavender oil
10 drops peppermint oil

Combine the lemon peel and rosemary leaves with the almond oil in a ceramic bowl. Stir the mixture vigorously with a wooden spoon and let it rest for five minutes. Put the mixture in a slow-cooking pot set at low, or place the oil and herbs in a covered ovenproof dish and bake in the oven at a very low heat (200° F) for three to four hours. When the mixture is cured, strain out the herbs and discard. Return the oil to a metal bowl and allow to cool to a tepid temperature. Add the oils of lavender and peppermint and stir the mixture with a metal spoon to combine. The oil should be yellow, with a strong green-citrus fragrance. Store the oil at room temperature in a labeled, lidded jar or plastic container for up to six months.

APPLICATION: Use the oil when you receive a full-body massage, head rubs, or foot rubs. If you can't afford or don't have time for massages, use the oil as per the Headache Head Rub (page 91). You can also add two tablespoonfuls of the oil to a hot bath.

Oily Hair ❧

Grease-Cutter Hair Rinse

———— ◄◦► ————

One of the principal features of a bad hair day is limp, dull, oily hair. Frequent washing with strong detergent shampoos causes your scalp to produce excess oil as a form of hair self-defense. If your hair is too oily, think about your diet. Just like your skin, your hair gets oily if you eat foods high in oil, sugar, salt, and saturated fat.

Years ago, women brushed powdered orris root through their hair to absorb and remove excess oil. It left the hair shiny, fluffy, clean, and sweet-smelling, but it was a very time-consuming process. Because of the convenience, hair rinses are nowadays all the rage. To cut through oily buildup on your hair and scalp, try the following hair-rinse recipe.

INGREDIENTS:
1 cup lemon juice
2 tablespoons grated lemon peel
1 cup rose water
10 drops lavender oil
10 drops rosemary oil

Put the lemon juice and rose water in a metal bowl and stir with a metal spoon until thoroughly combined. Add the lemon peel and stir again. Allow the mixture to sit at room temperature for three hours. Place a cheesecloth-lined strainer into a large bowl and pour the rinse into it. After the liquid drains into the bowl, gather the corners of the cheesecloth and squeeze the remaining liquid out of the grated lemon peel. Discard the cheesecloth. Add the oils of lavender and rosemary and stir with a metal spoon to combine. The rinse should be a tawny yellow color and smell beautifully of roses and lemons. This recipe is good for one use only. You may double or triple the recipe and refrigerate the rinse for future use. Discard any unused rinse after two weeks.

APPLICATION: Pour the rinse through your hair after washing with a mild shampoo. Vigorously massage the rinse into your hair and scalp. Catch the runoff in a bowl and repeat the procedure. Pour the rinse over your hair one final time, then wrap your head in a thick towel. Use the rinse twice a week, or until your hair and scalp can retain shine and body between shampooing.

NOTE: Conditioners, gels, and hair-mousse styling products can all leave a buildup on your hair. Reduce your use of these products if your hair is dull, oily, or unmanageable.

Oily Skin 🌿

Herbal Toner for Oily Skin

———— ◄◦► ————

If you like your food icky, sticky, gooey, or fried in deep fat, expect your skin to be oily. Excess oil is released through facial pores, enlarging them in the process and giving your complexion a shiny look. Junk food rampages also rob you of nutrition needed for radiant skin and other minor details, like a strong immune system. Though diet is the most important (and changeable) oily skin culprit, hormonal activity, stress, heredity, and nervous tension also contribute.

Eat more fruits, vegetables, and cooked grains if you want to take the shine off your nose. While you are experimenting with that, try using the following toner.

INGREDIENTS:
1½ cups commercial witch hazel extract
1 tablespoon grated lemon peel
1 tablespoon dried rosemary leaves
2 tablespoons dried comfrey root pieces
½ cup rose water
2 drops lavender oil
2 drops rosemary oil

Pour the witch hazel extract and rose water into a spotlessly clean quart-size jar with a tight-fitting lid. Shake the jar to combine the liquids, then add the remaining ingredients in the order given. Screw on the lid and shake the jar vigorously for five minutes. Label the jar with the date and name of the mixture, put it in a dark closet, and shake the jar for five minutes each day for the next two weeks. Decant the mixture by straining out the herbs through fine-weave cheesecloth. Wring all the liquid from the herbs before discarding them. The toner should be light brown, with a scent of roots and flowers. Return the toner to the labeled jar. Store the finished toner away from light and heat. Discard unused toner after six weeks and mix up a fresh batch.

APPLICATION: Apply a palmful of the toner to your cleansed face every night. You may apply the toner during the day by keeping it in a small spray bottle and giving yourself a spritz from time to time.

Sinusitis ❧

Echinacea and Goldenseal Sinus Tincture

———— ◄◉► ————

You'll know your sinuses are infected if your head feels like an overripe melon about to burst, your balance is off, your vision is blurred, and your sense of smell is completely gone. This charming condition also features a thick, yellowish nasal discharge, watery eyes with dark circles under them, and a sensation of internal pressure around your eyeballs and jaw.

Sinuses become infected because of poor diet, low immune resistance, allergies, smoking, or prolonged colds or flu. If you get frequent sinus infections, examine your environment also. Do you spend forty-plus hours a week in an airtight office building? If so, you may need to get out and take a brisk walk every day. Exercise is always good for what ails you, but especially so for sinus sufferers.

INGREDIENTS:
2 cups high-quality vodka
2 tablespoons goldenseal root powder
2 tablespoons echinacea root powder

Pour the vodka into a spotlessly clean quart-size jar with a tight-fitting lid. Add the remaining ingredients in the order given. Screw on the lid and shake the jar vigorously for five minutes. Label the jar with the date and name of the tincture, put it in a dark closet, and shake the jar for five minutes each day for the next two weeks. Decant the tincture by straining out the herbs through fine-weave cheesecloth. Discard the herbs and return the strained mixture to the labeled jar. Keep the finished tincture away from light and heat. Discard leftover tincture after one year and make a fresh batch if necessary.

APPLICATION: Give yourself ten to fifteen drops under the tongue four times each day, between meals, until the infection is gone. This tincture tastes nasty, so keep a warmed drink of milk or water on hand for a quick chaser.

NOTE: Use the Head Congestion Bath (page 89) for temporary relief from sinus congestion. The Headache Head Rub (page 91) is also good for relieving headache pain. If your sinus infection does not respond to treatment within four days, consult with a physician.

Skin Rashes 🦋

Skin Rash Bath Gel

———— ◀◦▶ ————

Itchy, scaly, flaky, rashy skin is very distressing, especially if you don't know what is causing it. Obvious
environmental allergens, such as poison oak and ivy,
create an immediately itchy rash upon contact, while
food allergies have a subtler, though no less irritating,
effect. Psoriasis and eczema are familiar skin-rash
conditions, but proven causes are still up for grabs.

Whatever is causing your skin to rash over, the
Skin Rash Bath Gel will help. Simply bathing in
warm water does loads of good, and the healing
herbs and oils contained in the gel will moisten,
purify, and heal your skin.

> INGREDIENTS:
> ½ cup finely ground oatmeal
> 1 cup olive oil
> 2 cups aloe vera gel
> 20 drops rosemary oil
> 20 drops lavender oil

Combine the oatmeal, olive oil, aloe vera gel, and
essential oils in a metal bowl. Stir the mixture with

a metal spoon until thoroughly mixed. The gel should be opaque and runny, like cake batter, with a smooth texture and strong rosemary scent. Run a comfortably warm bath. As the water is running, add the contents of the bowl to the tub, swirling the water with your hand until the oatmeal, gel, and oils are thoroughly combined. This mixture is good for one bath only.

APPLICATION: Soak in the bathtub for at least a half-hour. Do not wash with soap or rub your skin with a washcloth. Wet your hair with the bath-water, as the bath gel is also moisturizing and healing for your scalp and hair. When you are through soaking, rinse your body and hair in clear, warm water and allow your skin to air dry. Repeat the bath once each day until your skin rash improves and clears.

NOTE: Underlying nervous tension or food allergies are to be suspected if your rash is recurring or difficult to soothe. If your rash causes your skin to thicken, crack, or bleed, or if it starts to spread uncontrollably, consult with a body-oriented therapist, holistic practitioner, or dermatologist.

Sore Throats 🦋

Ginger and Goldenseal Gargle

———— ◄◦► ————

You are never so aware of how often you swallow until you have a sore throat. Then each little bite or sip causes you to pause and consider whether or not it is worth the effort. Luckily, you probably don't have much of an appetite anyway, except, of course, for therapeutic doses of ice cream.

Sore throats can be caused by strep infection, excessive smoking, colds, flu, or by screaming yourself hoarse at your kid's baseball game. Whatever has caused your throat to become sore, the Ginger and Goldenseal Gargle offers immediate relief.

INGREDIENTS:
2 cups water
1 tablespoon grated fresh ginger root
1/4 teaspoon powdered goldenseal root
1/4 cup lemon juice

Put the water in a covered pot and bring to a boil. Add the ginger root to the boiling water, cover the pot, and simmer for ten minutes. Remove the pot from the heat, add the powdered goldenseal root, and steep the mixture for ten more minutes. Thoroughly strain the liquid through fine-weave cheese-cloth or a coffee filter and discard the herbs. The liquid will be gold in color and should have no floating particles in it. Cool the gargle to a warm but comfortable gargling temperature before using. You may add honey or syrup to taste. This mixture is enough for two applications. Refrigerate the gargle and reheat with each use. Discard any remaining gargle after one day.

APPLICATION: Gargle with one cup of the liquid twice a day in the morning and evening until the soreness is relieved. If you have the nerve to gargle in the ladies room and you feel well enough to be up and about, put the gargle in a thermos and bring it to work with you.

NOTE: Small white spots in the back of the throat indicate a strep infection and should be examined by a physician. This gargle will not interfere with the action of prescribed antibiotics and can still be used as a throat soother. Persistent or chronic sore throats or sore throats accompanied by a fever higher than 101° may be symptoms of more serious underlying disorders. If you are experiencing any of these conditions, consult with a physician.

Stomachaches ❧

Tummy Trouble Tea

——— ◄◦► ———

Upset stomachs usually occur at the most inopportune times, as former president Bush can tell you. Stomachaches range from mild twinges to severe cramps, depending on the cause. Power lunches can upset your stomach because of the difficulty of relaxing and thoroughly digesting your meal while simultaneously dazzling your client, boss, or colleague. Constant eating-on-the-go has the same effect. Other tummy troublers are long-term nervous tension, cinched-in waists, and PMS.

Turbulent tummies require rest and relaxation first and foremost. The fast pace of modern life, however, often does not allow for R&R. If you often find yourself caught in board meetings, traffic jams, or various other vicious cycles, Tummy Trouble Tea will help.

INGREDIENTS:
2 drops rosemary oil
1/2 cup distilled culinary rose water
1 quart water

Heat the water in a covered pot until it is hot but not boiling. Remove from heat. Add the oil of rosemary and the rose water and stir the mixture with a metal spoon. Cool the tea to a comfortable drinking temperature before serving. Refrigerate the tea between servings and warm it for each use. Discard any unused tea after two days.

APPLICATION: Drink the tea as warm as you can stand, since heat can also help relieve stomachaches and cramps. Drink freely until symptoms disappear, usually after one or two cups. The tea has a pleasant taste and smell, though it may be sweetened with honey if you prefer. If you are on the go, pour the tea into a thermos and take a quick sip every now and then. Drinking a half-cup of the warm tea before eating can relax the stomach and help you to avoid further digestion trouble.

NOTE: Do not use this tea to relieve stomach upset caused by pregnancy. You may safely use Preggers Tea (page 103) for comparable results. If the stomachaches or cramps persist or grow worse, they may be a secondary effect of some other disorder. Consult with a physician for an accurate diagnosis and proper treatment.

Stretch Marks 🦋

Pregnant Breast and Belly Oil

——— ◄◦► ———

Your belly is the main focus of your own and everyone else's attention during your pregnancy, but don't forget that your breasts are expanding and are also vulnerable to stretch marks. As your skin expands, it will also itch. Moisturizing your skin with a nice rub relieves itching and forestalls stretch marks. Rubbing your belly also gives you and your growing baby a chance to get to know one another better.

Unfortunately, whether or not you will get stretch marks is largely a matter of heredity. If you prefer, however, not to leave these matters entirely up to your DNA, the following Pregnant Breast and Belly Oil may help.

INGREDIENTS:
1 cup extra-virgin olive oil
1 cup almond oil
2 tablespoons pearled barley
1 tablespoon organic rolled oats
1 tablespoon dried comfrey root pieces
20 drops lavender oil

Combine the olive oil, almond oil, barley, oats, and comfrey root pieces in a ceramic bowl. Stir the mixture with a wooden spoon and let it rest for five minutes. Put the mixture in a slow-cooking pot set at low, or place the oil and herbs in a covered ovenproof dish and bake in the oven at a very low heat (200° F) for three to four hours. When the mixture is cured, strain out and discard the herbs. The oil should be light brown in color, with a combined fragrance of grains and olive oil. Add the oil of lavender and stir the mixture with a metal spoon. Store the oil at room temperature in a labeled, lidded jar for up to six months.

APPLICATION: Place the glass jar containing the oil in a small pot of cold water. Warm the water until small bubbles form in the bottom of the pot. Remove the pot from the heat and pour a small amount of the warmed oil into your palm. Apply the warmed oil generously to your belly and breasts. Pay special attention to the area around your navel, the sides of your breasts, and the taut area between your belly and hip bones. Absorb excess oil with a soft towel when you are finished applying it. You may repeat the application as often as you like.

Swollen Glands 🦋

Swollen Gland Muffler

——— ◄◦► ———

Your lymphatic glands are usually just another invisible part of your internal self, until they become
swollen. Then they become soft, floating little marbles
of pain, turning each swallow into a memorable experience. These glands act as weather vanes for illness
and fill with lymphatic fluid in response to bacterial
or viral invasion, stress, smoking, or exhaustion.

Resting and drowning yourself in tea and juice is
a standard, and excellent, remedy for swollen
glands. To relieve pain and reduce swelling while
you are thus occupied, you may also use the following muffler.

> INGREDIENTS:
> 2 cups almond oil
> 1 ounce dried pennyroyal leaves
> 20 drops rosemary oil
> 20 drops peppermint oil
> long strip of clean flannel

Combine the pennyroyal leaves with the almond oil
in a ceramic bowl. Stir the mixture with a wooden

spoon and let it rest for five minutes. Put the mixture in a slow-cooking pot set at low, or place the oil and pennyroyal leaves in a covered ovenproof dish and bake in the oven at a very low heat (200° F) for three to four hours. When the mixture is cured, strain out and discard the pennyroyal leaves. Return the strained oil to a metal bowl. The oil should be pale yellow, with a strong camphor-mint fragrance. Add the oils of rosemary and peppermint and stir with a metal spoon until all the oils are combined. Store the oil at room temperature in a labeled, lidded jar or plastic container for up to six months.

APPLICATION: Purchase or prepare a clean strip of flannel 4 feet long and 1 foot wide. Gently rub a palmful of the oil into your throat, starting at the point of your jaw slightly behind the ears and continuing down to the collarbone. When the oil is applied and absorbed, warm the flannel strip in the dryer and wrap it around your throat. Leave the wrap on all night, tying it loosely in back to make sure you will sleep comfortably. In the morning, wash the unabsorbed oil off your throat and wash the flannel. Repeat the procedure once each night until the swelling recedes.

NOTE: If the swollen neck glands are intolerably painful or persist after one week of treatment, if you develop a fever (101° or higher), or if glandular swelling occurs anywhere else in the body, such as the armpit or groin, consult with a physician.

Vaginal Infections &

Plantain and Goldenseal Douche

———— ◄◦► ————

Your vagina maintains a delicate internal balancing act between acid and alkaline. When this balance is upset, formerly beneficial vaginal bacteria grow unchecked, resulting in a vaginal infection. Long-term stress, unlubricated sex, pregnancy, childbirth, and allergic reactions can all cause vaginal infections, as will systemic antibiotics, which mow down all bacteria, beneficial or otherwise. The following douche restores the proper vaginal pH, fights infection, and relieves the itching and burning sensation of a vaginal infection.

> INGREDIENTS:
> 2 ounces dried plantain leaves
> 2 tablespoons goldenseal root powder
> 1 tablespoon echinacea powder
> 1 quart water
> 2 drops lavender oil

Combine the plantain leaves, goldenseal root powder, powdered echinacea, and water in a covered pot and simmer for twenty minutes. Strain out the herbs through two layers of fine-weave cheesecloth or a coffee filter and discard. The mixture will be opaque and dark gray-green in color, with a pungent, grassy smell. Pour the mixture into a metal bowl and allow it to cool to a comfortable temperature. Add the oil of lavender and stir with a metal spoon to combine. This formula is enough for one application.

APPLICATION: If necessary, boil the douche bag and syringe before using to be completely certain they are sterile. Pour the cooled douche formula into the bag, adding enough plain water to fill it. Douche as you normally do, applying the formula to the interior vaginal environment, the vaginal lips, the perineum, and the anus. Use the entire contents of the douche bag. When finished, shower or bathe using an unscented, pH-balanced soap. Repeat the douche every other day until the infection is gone.

NOTE: Wear cotton panties when you have a yeast infection, as synthetic materials aggravate the condition. If you experience severe itching and discharge, put French green cosmetic clay on a panty liner and wear it throughout the day, changing the liner and the clay application every two hours.

Varicose Veins ❧

Varicose Vein Liniment

———◄◦►———

Unless you resemble a female Arnold Schwarze-
negger, your legs contain the biggest muscles and
veins in your body. When you walk, swim, or run,
these large muscles and veins pump quantities of
blood back to your heart for oxygenation. Little one-
way valves in the veins keep things moving in the
right direction, but these valves become sluggish if
you sit or stand all day, or if you are in the late
stages of pregnancy. Those familiar purple road
maps are really swollen veins filled with blood
waiting to complete the circuit.

Varicose veins are often hereditary, but exercise
and nutrition can make a big difference. While you
are organizing your exercise and nutrition plan, try
the following liniment.

INGREDIENTS:
2 cups commercial witch hazel tincture
1 tablespoon goldenseal root powder
1 tablespoon dried comfrey root pieces
2 tablespoons grated fresh ginger root
40 drops lavender oil

129

Pour the witch hazel tincture into a spotlessly clean quart-size jar with a tight-fitting lid. Add the remaining ingredients in the order given. Screw on the lid and shake the jar vigorously for five minutes. Label the jar with the date and name of the liniment, put it in a dark closet, and shake the jar for five minutes each day for the next two weeks. Decant the liniment by straining out the herbs through two layers of fine-weave cheesecloth. Discard the herbs and return the strained mixture to the labeled jar. Keep the finished liniment away from light and heat. With proper care, this liniment will keep indefinitely, becoming more effective with age.

APPLICATION: Lie comfortably on your back with pillows under your legs to elevate them. Be sure to protect bed linens or upholstery with a sheet or towel. Pour some liniment into your palm and rub vigorously, starting at your ankles and moving up your legs toward your heart. Perform this procedure once a day until aching and swelling subside. Though it cannot be guaranteed, varicose veins may start to fade as a result of this procedure.

Water Retention ❦

Diuretic Tea

———— ◄◦► ————

Increased estrogen levels cause water retention in muscle and connective tissues, which explains the bloated feeling many women get just before the monthly period. Hands, wrists, feet, and ankles may swell uncomfortably in the final months of pregnancy, for the same reason. Along with a puffy appearance, water retention also brings with it a feeling of hovering anxiety and nervousness, for reasons that are as yet unclear.

The best cure for water retention is to drink as much water as you can, which stimulates your kidneys and bladder to work harder at removing excess water from your system. The following diuretic tea will gently hasten this process.

INGREDIENTS:
½ cup pearled barley
1 quart water
1 tablespoon grated fresh ginger root
1 tablespoon dried plantain
1 teaspoon goldenseal root powder

Combine the barley and water in a large covered pot, bring to a boil, and simmer for forty minutes. Strain the mixture, reserving the cooked barley for breakfast or as a thickener in soup. Return the barley water to the pot and add the ginger root, plantain, and goldenseal. Bring the mixture to a boil and simmer for twenty minutes. Strain the mixture through a fine-mesh sieve and then again through a coffee filter until there are no floating particles. Discard the herbs. Return the brew to a bowl and allow it to cool to a tepid temperature. The brew will be opaque, with a grainy, grassy, gingery smell.

APPLICATION: Drink one cup of brew three times a day until results are achieved. You may add lemon juice and honey to taste. You may not like the taste of the tea; if so, have an organic cranberry juice chaser on hand each time you drink it. Refrigerate the brew between servings. Discard any unused brew after three days and make up a fresh batch if necessary.

NOTE: Do not use this tea during pregnancy. You may safely use the Preggers Tea recipe (page 103) for comparable results. If you are extremely uncomfortable or in pain due to swelling, consult with a holistic practitioner or physician.

Wrinkles 🏵

Rose Water, Lemon, and Almond Oil Facelift

———— ◄◦► ————

I read somewhere that wrinkles give you character, but I need a little more convincing, or possibly a little more character. Though I would never consider plastic surgery to remove wrinkles, I don't enjoy having them, and I devote considerable energy to keeping my fabulous face wrinkle-free. Squinting, frowning, sun exposure, smoking, and aging are all proven skin-wrinklers. Despite an ever-growing number of commercial creams on the market, each one claiming more miraculous skin-smoothing effects than the last, I will stick with the following soothing, reliable, wrinkle-removing routine.

INGREDIENTS:
2 cups almond oil
3 tablespoons grated lemon peel
¼ cup rose water
medium pot of hot water

Combine the almond oil and grated lemon peel in a slow-cooking pot set at low, or place the oil and lemon peel in a covered ovenproof dish and bake in the oven at a very low heat (200° F) for three to four hours. When the mixture is cured, strain out the lemon peel and discard. The oil should be tawny gold in color, with a delightful lemon smell. Pour the oil into a labeled glass jar and allow it to cool to a tepid temperature. Keep the oil in a cool cupboard or closet, away from heat and light. Discard after six months.

APPLICATION: Find a comfortable place for a face massage and arrange there the oil, rose water, and the pot of hot water with a small hand towel soaking in it. Massage a small amount of warmed oil into your face. Be sure to use an upward motion, starting with the delicate skin of the neck and gently moving upward to the roots of your hair and outward to your ears. Firmly rub the oil into any area of your face where there are established or newly formed wrinkles. When you have finished your facial massage and the oil is absorbed, apply a palmful of rose water to your face and neck. Lie back and apply the hot towel—after wringing most of the water out of it—to your face. When the towel cools, let it reheat in the pot of water while you apply more rose water to your face. Repeat this procedure until the rose water is gone. You can perform this relaxing ritual as often as you like to soften your wrinkles-in-residence and to keep new ones from forming. Although this procedure takes years off your appearance and feels wonderful, it is not guaranteed to completely remove or prevent wrinkles.

You now have at your disposal all the information you need to start preparing your Women's Home Remedy Kit. Enjoy your present and future preparations, explorations, and, hopefully, contributions to the healthful and flourishing world of herbs.

Part 3

Source Guide

Some Recommendations

I have found myself using the same herbs, equipment, and information sources over and over in my years as an herbalist. The reason for this is purely practical: my requests, whether for information or supplies, are promptly filled, usually with a pleasant phone conversation or reciprocal request for advice thrown in. Included in this final section of the book is a list of names, addresses, and phone numbers I recommend to help you meet your own herb and information needs.

From the hundreds of possible herb and essential oil suppliers, herb farms, and herbal bath and body shops throughout the nation, I have selected my ten favorites to start you off. All of these businesses fulfill my list of essentials for an herb supplier: they charge reasonable prices, they are stable businesses, they provide a large selection of herbs, oils, equipment, and other delightful products for you to enjoy, and they will politely and promptly fill your order. Most of them take wholesale or retail orders, and some wholesale suppliers will fill orders of as little as one pound of a particular herb.

My selection of herb publications was based on the following criteria: the publication is representative of a national organization for herbalists, it provides the latest medicinal, chemical, legal, or cosmetic research and information on herbs and essential oils both in the United States and abroad, and it provides regular editorial contributions by well-known and respected herbalists. Most include herbal calendars of events, lists of recommended herb schools and universities, and referrals to holistic MDs, homeopaths, and practicing herbalists. The quality of illustration, layout, and design also influenced my decision, but beyond a certain level of organization, I did not consider these elements to be essential.

Wholesale and Retail
Mail-Order Outlets

———— ◄◌► ————

Aphrodisia
Joanne Pelletier
264 Bleecker Street
New York, NY 10014
(212) 989-6440

Bulk herbs, essential oils, bath products, tea blends, herb tinctures.

Avena Botanicals
Deb Soule
20 Mill Street
Rockland, ME 04841
(207) 594-0694

Herb tinctures and extracts, formulas, tea blends, herbal creams, herbal oils.

Devonshire Apothecary
Nancy "J.J." Levy
P.O. Box 160215
606 Blanco, Pecan Square
Austin, TX 78703
(512) 477-8270

Dried botanicals and spices, tea blends, herb tinctures, body products, essential oils.

Frontier Cooperative Herbs
Rick Stewart, C.E.O.
Box 299
Norway, IA 52318
(800) 786-1388

Bulk organic herbs, body products, tea blends, essential oils.

Gaia Botanicals
Lorna Bradley
P.O. Box 8485
Philadelphia, PA 19101
(215) 222-5499

Bulk herbs, floral waters, beeswax candles.

Great Lakes Herb Company
Ron Holch
P.O. Box 6713
Minneapolis, MN 55406
(612) 486-2595

Organic bulk herbs, essential oils, tinctures, herb capsules, body products.

Hausmann's Pharmacy, Inc.
Irene Paul
534–536 W. Girard Avenue
Philadelphia, PA 19123
(800) 235-5522

Herbs, herb extracts, bath oils, essential oils, herbal tea blends.

Herb-Pharm
P.O. Box 116
Williams OR 97544
(503) 846-6262

Single and compound herbal tinctures, small selection of bulk herbs.

Mountain Rose Herbs
Julie Bailey
P.O. Box 2000
Redway, CA 95560
(800) 879-3337

Bulk herbs, beverage teas and blends, equipment for herbal preparations, body products, herbal extracts.

Nature's Herb
Emma Beattie
1010 46th Street
Emeryville, CA 94608
(510) 601-0700

Bulk herbs, essential oils, tea blends.

Herbal Publications and Newsletters

——— ◄◌► ———

American Botanical Council
P.O. Box 201660
Austin, TX 78720-1660
(512) 331-8868

Research reviews from scientific literature, legal issues, market trends, media coverage of herbs.

NEHA
The Northeast Herbal Association
P.O. Box 146
Marshfield, VT 05658-0146
(802) 479-9825

Feature articles, event calendars, medical topics,
legal updates, supply sources.

The Herb Companion
Interweave Press
201 East 4th Street
Loveland, CO 80537
(303) 669-7672

Bimonthly magazine covering national and interna-
tional herb lore, herbs for weddings, preserving
herbs, soaps.

The Herbal Green Pages
The Herb Growing and Marketing Network
P.O. Box 245
Silver Springs, PA 17575-0245
(717) 393-3295

Information on wholesale and retail outlets, equipment suppliers, gardens, organic information.

The Herb Quarterly
P.O. Box 689
San Anselmo, CA 94960-9801
(415) 455-9540

Herbal updates, book reviews, herb profiles, recipes, calendars of herbal events.

Herb Research Foundation
1007 Pearl Street, Suite 200
Boulder, CO 80302
(303) 449-2265

Research reviews from scientific literature, legal issues, market trends, media coverage of herbs.

The Herbalist
The Herb Society of America
9019 Kirtland-Chardon Road
Mentor, OH 44060
(216) 256-0514

Annual journal of the Herb Society of America. Articles on all aspects of herbs written by HSA members.

The Herb, Spice, and Medicinal Plant Digest
Lyle E. Craker
Department of Plant & Soil Sciences
University of Massachusetts
Amherst, MA 01003
(413) 545-2347

News about herbs in medicinal research, important people in the herb world, herbs and chemistry, reviews of the herb literature.